CURRENT PERSPECTIVES IN CULTURAL PSYCHIATRY

CURRENT PERSPECTIVES IN CULTURAL PSYCHIATRY

Edited by

Edward F. Foulks
Department of Psychiatry
University of Pennsylvania

Ronald M. Wintrob
Depts. of Psychiatry and Anthropology
University of Connecticut

Joseph Westermeyer
Department of Psychiatry
University of Minnesota

Armando R. Favazza
Department of Psychiatry
University of Missouri-Columbia

S P Books Division of
SPECTRUM PUBLICATIONS, INC.
New York

Distributed by Halsted Press
A Division of John Wiley & Sons

New York   Toronto   London   Sydney

SPECTRUM PUBLICATIONS, INC.
175-20 Wexford Terrace, Jamaica, N.Y. 11432

Library of Congress Cataloging in Publication Data

Main entry under title:

Current perspectives in cultural psychiatry.

Includes index.
1. Psychiatry, Transcultural. I. Foulks, Edward F.
RC455.4.E8C87   616.8'9   77-22797
ISBN 0-89335-027-3

Distributed solely by the Halsted Press Division of John Wiley & Sons, Inc.
New York, New York
ISBN 0-470-99176-3

Contributors

MORLEY BEISER, M.D.
Department of Psychiatry
University of British Columbia
Vancouver, British Columbia

OTTO BILLIG, M.D.
Department of Psychiatry
Vanderbilt University
Nashville, Tennessee

PATRICIA BUFFLER, M.S.
University of Alaska
Anchorage, Alaska

B. G. BURTON-BRADLEY, M.D.
Chief of the Division of
   Mental Health Services
Papua New Guinea Government
Papua, New Guinea

ARMANDO FAVAZZA, M.D., M.P.H.
Department of Psychiatry
University of Missouri
Columbia, Missouri

EDWARD F. FOULKS, M.D., Ph.D.
Departments of Psychiatry
   and Anthropology
University of Pennsylvania
Philadelphia, Pennsylvania

DESMOND FUNG, M.D.
Department of Psychiatry
Cedars Sinai Hospital
Los Angeles, California

WALTER GOLDSCHMIDT, Ph.D.
Department of Anthropology
University of California
Los Angeles, California

EZRA GRIFFITH, M.D.
Department of Psychiatry
Yale University
   School of Medicine
New Haven, Connecticut

EARLINE HOUSTON, M.D.
Department of Psychiatry
Hahnemann Medical College
   and Hospital
Philadelphia, Pennsylvania

MAMORU IGA, Ph.D.
Department of Sociology
California State University
Northridge, California

ARI KIEV, M.D.
Department of Psychiatry
Cornell University
New York, New York

ROBERT F. KRAUS, M.D.
Department of Psychiatry
University of Washington
Seattle, Washington

JULIA LAM, M.D.
Department of Psychiatry
University of Southern California
School of Medicine
Los Angeles, California

MARY OMAN, M.A.
Department of Anthropology
University of Missouri
Columbia, Missouri

MANSELL PATTISON, M.D.
Department of Psychiatry
University of California, Irvine
Irvine, California

MARGARET PERRY, M.S.
Department of Psychiatry
University of Missouri
Columbia, Missouri

PEDRO RUIZ, M.D.
Department of Psychiatry
Albert Einstein College of Medicine
Bronx, New York

JOHN SCHWAB, M.D.
Department of Psychiatry
Louisville University
School of Medicine
Louisville, Kentucky

MARY SCHWAB, M.D.
Massachusetts Mental Health Center
Boston, Massachusetts

JAMES SHORE, M.D.
Department of Psychiatry
University of Oregon
Portland, Oregon

CHOMCHAN SOUNDALAY, M.D.
Director, National
Detoxification Center
Vientiene, Laos

JOHN P. SPIEGAL, M.D.
The Florence Heller Graduate
School for Advanced Studies in
Social Welfare
Brandeis University
Waltham, Massachusetts

FRANK TAN, M.D.
Department of Psychiatry
Cedars Sinai Hospital
Los Angeles, California

JAMES WEISS, M.D., M.P.H.
Department of Psychiatry
University of Missouri
Columbia, Missouri

JOSEPH WESTERMEYER, M.D.,
Ph.D.
Department of Psychiatry
University of Minnesota
Minneapolis, Minnesota

RONALD WINTROB, M.D.
Department of Psychiatry
University of Connecticut
Farmington, Connecticut

JOE YAMAMOTO, M.D.
Department of Psychiatry
University of Southern California
Los Angeles, California

Contents

Part II—CURRENT RESEARCH IN CULTURAL PSYCHIATRY IN THE UNITED STATES

Part III—CROSS-CULTURAL RESEARCH BY AMERICAN PSYCHIATRISTS OUTSIDE OF NORTH AMERICA

Acknowledgments

As senior editor I would like to pay tribute to the efforts of Doctors Wintrob, Westermeyer, and Favazza. Each played a big role in the original organization of subjects and contributors at the Annual Meeting of the American Psychiatric Association which was held in May 1976 in Miami. At that meeting, four scientific panels were devoted to the subject of cultural psychiatry. The panels were headed by each of our editors respectively. The ordering of the editors' names on this volume in no way reflects the degree of their contribution; instead, names are ordered according to the logical sequence contained in the subject of this book.

Edward F. Foulks, M.D., Ph.D.

Introduction

JOHN P. SPIEGEL

This is an important book. The reader, however, may experience some initial difficulty in determining just where to place it within the broad parameters of the profession of psychiatry.

It is generally assumed that the study of mental health and illness is based on the distinction between biological, psychological and social determinants of pathology. Models of the treatment of psychiatric disorders are based on a similar, tripartite distinction, and the well-trained therapist is expected to be familiar with all three of these contributory factors. If the term "Social Psychiatry" roughly covers the relation of social and environmental factors to the causation and treatment of mental illness, then what is meant by "Cultural Psychiatry?" Does it refer to a sub-specialty within the broader area of social psychiatry? If so, what are the boundaries of the sub-specialty?

Questions of this order are not directly addressed by the editors or their contributors. In fact, the title and its subject matter, cultural psychiatry, remain largely undefined. This is not said in a spirit of criticism. The presumably more comprehensive field of social psychiatry has experienced the same lack of definition over a period of many years.[1] Furthermore, there is a certain advantage in keeping a developing field open, loose, even vague. The lack of boundaries functions as a wel-come-to-the-club signal and the growth of the field is thereby promoted. The determination of what is central to a field, as distinguished from peripheral or subordinate issues, can come later when a larger number of professionals have established themselves and the resulting literature is ready for codification.

From this point of view, the present volume is something of a paradox. The editors very clearly perceive cultural psychiatry as the continuation in a new key of an honorable tradition: The historical collaboration be-tween anthropology and psychiatry. In Chapter 1, "Anthropology and Psychiatry: A New Blending of an Old Relationship," Edward Foulks dates the interface between the two disciplines from the publication of Freud's *Totem and Taboo* in 1914. In Chapter 2, Walter Goldschmidt moves the association back to "the very birth of anthropology," through the influence of the psychologist, Wilhelm Wundt, on the anthropologist, Franz Boas. Following the law of expanding boundaries, the Schwabs, in Chapter 18, "The Future of Cultural Psychiatry," trace a scholarly interest in culture and mental illness back to the early decades of the 19th century. And, as to the quantity of publications, in Chapter 3, Armando Favazza and Mary Oman report on their codification of 3,624 articles in the area of cultural psychiatry published since 1925—a Her-culean task in itself.

From the perspective of this long history of association between the two professions, one may ask what is new about this "New Blending of an Old Relationship?" Also, why is a new blending necessary? What was wrong with the old, established blend?

The editors and their contributors propose answers to these ques-tions. To begin with, the relationship between psychiatry and anthro-pology has always been unstable and subject to unexpected changes, a natural enough condition considering the changing character of the question of method. The "old blend" was heavily weighted with theory, especially psychoanalytically-based theory. The theoretical assumptions were often constructed *a priori* and they were applied to data drawn from secondary sources, as in the case of *Totem and Taboo*. The search was for cultural universals which could be applied to psychodynamics and for psychoanalytic universals which could be applied in anthro-pology, usually within an evolutionary perspective. Nevertheless, the outcome of this partnership in the culture-and-personality studies, with their focus on differences in child-rearing patterns in different cultures, despite its somewhat questionable methods, did firmly establish the relevance of each discipline for the other. Still, the question of the pay-off from this partnership for therapeutic goals was never really resolved.

The new emphasis stresses the collection of primary data, in the field, and with a clinical focus. As if to underscore this point, all but one of the senior authors in the present volume is a clinician. Psychiatrists as providers of service, it would seem, are assuming a dominant role in the partnership. Thus: "Cultural Psychiatry."

If the codification of the voluminous but disbursed literature of the past has led to no particular "breakthrough"—and according to Favazza and Oman it has not—then perhaps the source of the difficulty was too much theory and not enough attention to concrete observation. Theoretical variation gave rise to controversy and the subsequent search for data to reinforce one or another theoretical position. The new approach does not ignore theory but holds it at a respectful distance while insisting on the need for the clinician to do research and the researcher to pursue therapeutic goals. This combination of skills requires that the cultural psychiatrist become familiar *in depth* with patients in a culture other than his own. To obtain detailed knowledge at this level the clinician must work for a considerable period of time in the field, exposing him-self as a stranger to strange experiences, learning how to perceive health and illness from the standpoint of the novel perspectives, values and conceptualizations of a culture other than his own. In short, in his preparation and training for the delivery of services, he must undergo the field experiences of the anthropologist.

These are the general explanations of the "new blend" proposed by the editors. To me, their descriptions of cultural psychiatry appear cor-rect and pertinent. But their general formulations do not exhaust the range of particular concerns to be found in this book. The contributors have presented a number of subsidiary issues which, while not al-together new, provide a hard-edged clinical approach to the long association between anthropology and psychiatry—one that is pointedly consistent with a number of contemporary themes in science and in the world. The themes are related to each other and to the principles of cultural psychiatry presented by the editors. In what follows, I shall give a brief account of these more concrete issues. However, no attempt will be made to systematize or integrate the issues.

One of these themes is the need to be aware of and appropriately responsive to the polyethnic characteristics of contemporary societies. The issue goes further than the recent emphasis given to "cultural pluralism." It goes beyond "Beyond the Melting Pot," beyond sen-sitivity to the rights and needs of minorities. It is concerned with the relation of cultural groups and subgroups to each other as well as to the dominant group at the top of the hierarchy of political control. From this point of view, there is little difference between modernizing societies emerging from colonialism in Africa and Asia and the fully-developed societies of the West. For example, in Chapter 6, James Shore discusses the role of the clinician in helping the native American population to distinguish between the health and illness patterns of different Indian tribes. Contrary to the general belief held even by tribal leaders, namely the general stereotype of the suicidal Indian, research has shown that high rates of suicide are restricted to certain rapidly acculturating Alaskan natives and Northern Great Plains groups. As Shore states, a non-Indian "Anglo" misconception had become incorporated as an Indian belief, with the accompanying loss of self-esteem and a blocking of rational preventive health planning.

In Chapter 6 Walter Goldschmidt describes the different ways in which initiation ceremonies and witchcraft accusations are used among four closely related African subgroups as a defense against the stress of switching from a pastoral to a farming economy and finally applies such "institutional defenses" to the behavior of the student radicals of the '60's. In Chapter 9, Ronald Wintrob compares beliefs in the supernatural causes of illness, including mental illness, among Blacks (Rootwork,) Puerto Ricans (Espiritismo) and Whites belonging to Pentecostal and other fundamentalist Christian sects (Faith Healing.) No evidence is presented that these similar belief systems among different ethnic populations have influenced each other, though in my opinion this may well have happened in the remote past. In all these instances, the polyethnic perspective embraces both the *similarities* and the *differences* among the institutional stresses and defenses associated with mental illness among various widely dispersed or closely related sub-cultural groups.

A related issue is concerned with the tremendous amount of borrowing and lending of cultural traits across ethnic boundaries—with both pathological and therapeutic results! How ethnic groups maintain their boundaries and their sense of identity in the face of such exchanges of cultural traits—often labelled "acculturation"—has been illuminated by Barth[2] and his collaborators.[3] In the present volume, the pathological effects of cultural borrowing are illustrated in Burton-Bradley's discussion in Chapter 13 of "Cannibalism for Cargo." Cargo cults in Melanesian societies arise in circumstances wherein a preliterate group based on a very simple technology encounters a highly developed, materialistic culture based on a complex technology. Under conditions of increasing deprivation, such preliterate groups develop "Cargo Thinking," a magical belief system based on the expectation that one of their ancestor spirits or gods will deliver the material riches and power of the complex socity, (the "Cargo,") under the sponsorship of a local, charismatic leader, on a day of great, cataclysmic changes. The problem is that the belief systems arising from traditional rituals become infiltrated with ideas borrowed from the Old and New Testaments, spread by the teachings of Christian missionaries. In the case discussed by Burton-Bradley, a Papuan native of the traditionally cannibalistic Geilale tribe, basing himself on a misinterpretation of the Abraham-Isaac story, sacrificed his son and cannibalized parts of his son's body, in the hope that he would thereby become a Cargo Cult leader. The question of whether this behavior was culturally appropriate or deviant was resolved in favor of the latter by the patient's own kinsmen as well as other members of his group. The cultural borrowing and mixing was not the primary cause of the patient's pathology but it was a necessary, contributory factor.

On the positive side, cultural borrowing is associated with the possibility that ethnic groups traditionally employing supernatural concepts of illness can respond adaptively to the explanations and procedures of Western scientific medicine. Three papers in this collection discuss the clinical possibilities of combining traditional and Western perspectives on illness. They all emphasize the difficult but promising role of the clinician in working within such combinations of presumably incompatible cultural practices. In Chapter 8, on "Hex and Possession," Ruiz and Griffiths discuss the possibility of clinical experimentation with the "de-hexing" of a variety of psychosomatic and psychiatric symptoms by native healers. In Chapter 9, on "Beliefs and Behavior in the Treatment of Mental Illness," Wintrob describes the division of labor between native healers and clinicians, both working with a variety of ethnic groups and religious sects. The mix of beliefs can be handled because, for these subcultural groups certain medical conditions with an imern medicine while illnesses raising the question of remote cause ("Why medicine while illnesses raising the question of remote cause ("Why should this happen to me?") make concepts of malign intervention or spirit possession more suitable for traditional, supernatural cures. In Chapter 15, "An Addiction Treatment Program in Laos," Joseph Westermayer reveals that elderly, long-term opium addicts, displaying behavior traditionally accepted within the culture, were nevertheless able to respond to a methadone detoxification program, the principles of which were learned only on arrival at the treatment center.

In many instances, the borrowing, exchanging and mixing of cultural practices across ethnic boundaries does not occur. The nature of the conditions under which such exchanges can take place or are blocked require more research. But when the exchange is blocked in respect to Western psychiatric or psychological concepts, the qualifications on the provision of care by the clinician are severe. The outcomes of such rejection are described in the two papers by Joe Yamamoto: Chapter 10 on "Chinese-Speaking Vietnamese Refugees in Los Angeles," and Chapter 16 on "An Asian View of the Future of Cultural Psychiatry."

The themes of blocking, rejection, restriction or modification of the work of North American, scientifically-trained professionals are vividly presented in the chapters on research by James Shore ("Psychiatric Research Issues with American Indians") and by Morton Beiser ("Ethics in Cross-Cultural Research.") Whatever word one uses for the encounter between groups of widely varying lifestyles—"intercultural," "cross-cultural," or "transcultural"—the central process is concerned with a matching, a goodness- or badness-of-fit, between the concepts and practices of the two groups. Attention to this issue is one of the chief differences between the "old blend" and the "new blend" adopted in this book. In the era of Western Imperialism, with its colonial policies enforced by superior strength, researchers from the academic establishments in the West did not have to be too concerned about whether their work was wanted by their "native" research subjects or by the groups to which they belonged. Nor did they have to be concerned about who would benefit from their research. A possible contribution to Science was justification enough for the time, the money and the effort contributed by the professionals and by their subjects.

In the new perspectives of cultural psychiatry, these comfortable assumptions are viewed as irrelevant, embarrassing or possibly damaging. On the side of the "subjects" of research, populations, whether based on ethnicity, religion, race, class or sex, insist on determining for themselves whether the research is necessary or in their self-interest. The self-interest in question has two related aspects—one political and the other concerned with services. Having in the past so often felt exploited, put down, or used for the benefit of the researcher, cultural groups are determined to show that they now have the political power and the sophistication to control what research would be done. Because their needs are usually intense, the cultural groups demand that the outcome of any research result in improved services or the relief of distress. Research, in other words, must have a concrete and fairly immediate pay-off. A possible benefit in the distant future is treated with distinct skepticism. Thus even a health survey to determine needs on which to base future planning for services may receive low acceptance if more immediate and obvious needs have a higher perceived priority. And this priority may be assigned primarily on political grounds.

For the researcher, the contemporary premises create a negotiating or bargaining situation in which his sense of responsibility is increasingly tested. He must be able to make a convincing case that his research is relevant and beneficial. In addition, he must convince himself and the group that it will not harm the group as a whole nor any individuals who participate. This issue goes beyond the contemporary ethical and legal concerns with confidentiality, invasion of privacy and informed consent. The trouble is that the harm may come about in unanticipated ways. Beiser's chapter demonstrates that despite his observance of all the precautions of which he was aware, his research in Senegal was upsetting to the subjects because they were not able to understand the meaning of a "random sample," or of the concept of "chance." Neither did the concept of the individual *qua* individual have any meaning for the group. Everything that happens to an individual is attributed to natural or supernatural forces and reflects upon the group. The research which was simply concerned with health needs nevertheless aroused expectations of relief from illness and other stresses. When subjects who had been singled out randomly subsequently became ill in the usual run of illnesses, the researchers were held responsible and blamed for harming the group.

Other contributors address the issue of responsibility for culturally appropriate therapeutic or research interventions from a different angle of approach, for example, Chapter 14 on "Folk Healing in Suriname." A most extensive review of the mandate for intervention in different arrangements of private and public networks occurs in Mansell Pattison's "A Theoretical-Empirical Base for Social Systems Therapy" (Chapter 17.)

Despite the extensive coverage of these particular issues in the individual chapters, the book does not contain all the themes which might be included in a volume on Cultural Psychiatry. For example, there is no discussion of the provision of services to the broad spectrum of white ethnics in the United States[4,5] nor to the Black or Hispanic populations. Nor is consideration given to the modification of specific therapeutic modalities such as psychoanalysis[6] or behavior therapy[7] for the values of particular subcultural groups. But this book does not set out to be an encyclopaedia nor a comprehensive textbook. For its stated purpose—to spell out the principal characteristics of Cultural Psychiatry in the late '70's—the book deserves to be read with careful attention. Based on the accomplishments so far, one can look forward eagerly to further progress in this field. One can even hope that in the future all psychiatrists will become aware of the cultural aspects of their clinical work.

REFERENCES

1. Bell, Norman W. and John P. Spiegel. "Social Psychiatry: Vagaries of a Term," from *Archives of General Psychiatry*, Volume 14, April 1966.
2. Barth, Fredrik, (ed.) *Ethnic Groups and Boundaries*. Results of a symposium held at the University of Bergen, 23–26 February, 1967. Published in Boston by Little, Brown & Company, 1969.
3. Despres, Leo A. (ed.) *Ethnicity: Resource Competition in Plural Societies*. The Hague: Multon, 1975. Distributed in the United States by Aldine Books, Chicago.
4. Papajohn, John and John Spiegel. *Transactions in Families: A Modern Approach for Resolving Cultural and Generational Conflicts*. San Francisco: Jossey-Bass, Inc., 1975.
5. Giordano, Joseph. *Ethnicity and Mental Health*. National Project on Ethnic America of the American Jewish Committee, New York, 1976 (4th printing.)
6. Spiegel, John P. "Cultural Aspects of Transference and Countertransference Revisited," in *Journal of the American Academy of Psychoanalysis*, 4 (4): John Wiley & Sons, Inc., 1976, pp. 447–467.
7. Flannery, Raymond B., Jr. "Ethnicity in the Behavior Treatment of a Socially Isolated Adult," paper submitted for publication to *Psychotherapy: Theory, Research and Practice*, 1977.

Part I
ANTHROPOLOGICAL THEORY IN PSYCHIATRY

Introduction

EDWARD F. FOULKS

This section brings together the work of psychiatrists and anthropologists who have had an active interest in anthropological theory as it relates to issues current in psychiatry both in our country and abroad. Work in the field has proved a valuable testing ground for hypotheses of human behavior and its maladaptations, which have been formulated within the confines of Western society and Western cultural values. Many ideas basic to psychoanalytic psychology, psychiatric symptomotology, and epidemiological patterns of mental illnesses in other areas of the world continue to be of major concern. Psychiatry has for years been cognizant of the role of social change and social breakdown in such illnesses as alcoholism and other addictive diseases, hysteria, suicide and homocide, and depression. With the rapid development of Third-World nations come the problems of delivering adequate mental health services. The importance of developing diagnostic methods and therapeutic approaches to people of various ethnic backgrounds has been a continuing area of interface between anthropology and psychiatry, particularly in urban community mental health programs and in public health service programs for native populations. The training of various ethnic peoples, such as health aid programs and psychiatric education programs with folk healers, exemplifies such cooperative effort. Social factors involved in mental disorders have been recognized and have given rise to such approaches in psychiatry as family therapy, social-network therapy, and community organization.

This section explores some of these issues and others which are currently of great relevance not only to "cultural psychiatrists" but to the field of psychiatry as a whole. Chapter 1 by Edward Foulks details historical aspects of the relation between anthropology and psychoanalysis. Walter Goldschmidt, an anthropologist noted for his work on culture and personality, further outlines the historical development between the fields and carries his analysis to the present. Armando Favazza and Mary Oman have reviewed the mental health literature that makes reference to cross-cultural theory. Their effort is enlightening for it indicates how extensive and relevant the relation between the fields has been.

Ari Kiev outlines current issues in delivering mental health care to Third-World peoples, a subject of great relevance to cultural psychiatry today. Finally, James Weiss and Margaret Perry detail cultural problems encountered in defining and managing disordered behavior across cultural and social-class boundaries.

1

Anthropology and Psychiatry: A New Blending of an Old Relationship

EDWARD F. FOULKS

Cultural psychiatry is not new. The collaboration between anthropologists and psychiatrists and the application of anthropological theory to questions of psychiatric diagnosis, etiology, and treatment has gone on for more than half a century. This book thus represents the continuation of a tradition of mutual collaboration between the disciplines of anthropology and psychiatry.

As in other areas of psychiatry, discoveries through the years have culminated in approaches that today increasingly rely on an empirical base. Cultural psychiatry has evolved from the realm of the theoretical to a firmer grounding in data collected by scientific methods. We feel that this volume represents the most recent approaches of psychiatrists in North America and several other areas of the world who are investigating the problems of their patients from a cultural-psychiatric perspective. The book reflects much of what is currently going on among psychiatrists in America who are working in this field.

Early in this century a number of psychiatrists, most notably Freud and Jung, were interested in finding evidence that certain psychological complexes of man were universal. Freud discovered the unconscious and equated the primitive mental mechanisms of this realm of the mind with the way that "primitive people" actually thought and behaved. In a sense, he advocated that ontogeny recapitulates phylogeny by arguing that the mental life of the modern child parallels the steps in the evolution of society; and that civilization represents the ultimate repression and sublimation of the host of primitive impulses. The mind of the child, the mind of the neurotic, and the minds of primitive people were thus felt to be equivalent in some sense.

Freud's most serious foray into utilizing anthropological sources to substantiate his ideas is found in "Totem and Taboo" (1). This work created much controversy among anthropologists, and has become a classic reference of the ambivalence then accorded psychiatry by anthropologists. Freud argued that the Oedipus complex is to be found universally in all humans because it is part of our biological heritage. He pointed out that the totem is a symbolic representative of an ancestor to whom one has very special obligations. One such obligation is that the living representatives of the totem may not be killed or eaten; another is exogamy, that is, all male members of the totem must marry women from another lineage. Freud argued that the origin of this "primitive" social system was to be found in actual events in prehistory. In this primordial time, the patriarch had possession of the females. His sons, with their incestuous wishes for their mothers, overthrew the father, killed and ate him. So great was their guilt over this heinous crime that they forgot or repressed their incestuous desires and attempted to expiate their sins against the father by ritually identifying with him. Interestingly, such ritual identification took the form of symbolically eating the patriarch's flesh. Thus, argues Freud, in the primordial, primitive period of human evolution there was an actual situation whose impact on humans and society was of such magnitude as to become an inevitable inheritance of us all. Jung included the Oedipus complex in the realm of the collective unconscious and felt that it is one of the universal human archetypical patterns handed down from previous generations.

Anthropologists were disturbed by Freud's inappropriate use of unscientific anthropological references and perhaps even more by the implicit racist and ethnocentric notions contained in these ideas. Perhaps somewhat in response, the anthropologists of the 1920's and 1930's emphasized the principles of cultural relativism and explicitly eschewed Western European ethnocentrism.

In 1934 Ruth Benedict published her now famous book *Patterns of Culture* (2). The work culminated years of study with one of the founders of American anthropology, Franz Boas, at Columbia University and extensive fieldwork of her own in the southwestern United States among the Zuni, the Dobu of the South Pacific, and the Northwest Coast Kwakiutl Indians. She pointed out that in each society there is to be found a major organizing principle which she termed "ethos." Ethos, she felt, is derived from certain aspects of basic human temperament. The ethos of the Zuni is described as Apollonian. They are said to be unemotive, stoic, steadily ritualistic, orderly, not given to excesses, and to have solved the problems of living through rational processes rather than ecstatic inspiration. The Apollonian ethos permeates their architecture, their agricultural techniques, their household patterns, their child-rearing practices, their dances, artwork, and personalities. In contrast, Benedict believed that the Kwakiutl and most other North American Indian groups manifest a Dionysian ethos. They are described as being highly excitable, emotive, impulsive, prone to altered states of consciousness, and as seeking the solution of problems in ecstatic or frenzied states of mind. The spirit quest, as well as highly charged grandiose displays of potlatching, are cited as evidence supporting this thesis.

In reference to psychiatry, Benedict noted that American psychiatrists must assume an attitude of defining normal and abnormal only within the peculiar cultural context of the society they are investigating. There is no "normal" and there is no absolute "psychopathological." A normal Zuni would clearly be aberrant in Kwakiutl society, and conversely a normal Kwakiutl would be quite aberrant among the Zuni. Benedict felt that in every society individuals are born somewhere on a normal distribution curve of human temperament. Some individuals would be born, for example, with little aggression; most with moderate aggression; and a few with extreme aggression. Furthermore, the predominant ethos of a society is instilled throughout life in the individual by various socializing methods; thus, aspects of temperament may be learned. In Plains Indian society, mildly aggressive males do learn extremely aggressive displays. On the other hand, she argued, a few individuals may be temperamentally so far from the ideal ethos, that they cannot learn to participate in normal society. Therefore various phenomena would be considered abnormal, aberrant, or psychopathological. In the case of the Plains Indians, the aggression demanded of young males was so extreme that many were unable to meet these standards. Considering them abnormal and ostracizing or curing them would thus be ineffective.

So extreme was the Plains Indian ethos that an antithetical institution was created as a functional repository for those not up to the rigorous "Sun Dance" and other initiation rites. This institution was the "berdache." Here a male would assume the identity of a female and therefore avoid the extremes of aggression demanded of men. Benedict stressed throughout that the life of the "primitive" is not to be equated with the life of the neurotic. In fact, there is no absolute standard for diagnosing neurosis or psychosis. Instead, she cautioned psychiatrists about developing universal notions and applying them to all mankind.

Benedict's companion at Columbia University, Margaret Mead, also questioned universalistic theories proposed by Western European and American psychiatrists, and wrote a number of books which have since become classics. In each of these early works, Mead attacked a major shibboleth of American psychiatric theory.

In *Coming of Age in Samoa* (3), first published in 1928, Mead attacked the notion that adolescence is inevitably hallmarked by rebellion, emotional upheaval, and an inability to modulate the newly budding impulses and desires of puberty. Mead lived for nine months in Samoa, and she concluded that in this society adolescence is not a conflictual, rebellious period as in the West. She postulated that adolescent turmoil is not a biological inevitability, but instead is based on social configurations. More specifically, she argued that adolescent turmoil results from a discontinuity of roles between children and adults. Furthermore, in societies where continuities exist between what children and what adults do, there is no upheaval shortly after puberty. She pointed out that the facts of life and sex are not taboo subjects of conversation or behavior for young Samoan girls, and that in Samoa the transition into adulthood is smooth and long-developing. In contrast, she pointed out that in American society no gradual transition exists. Instead, suddenly and abruptly a girl becomes a "woman." She believed such discontinuity naturally results in considerable conflict.

Perhaps her most significant and forward-thinking early work was *Sex and Temperament in Three Primitive Societies* (4). Here, Mead studied three contiguous but culturally different New Guinea societies: the Mountain Arapesh, the river-dwelling Mundugumor, and the lake-dwelling Tchambuli. In her fieldwork among these people, Mead discovered that the stereotypes commonly held in the West regarding the temperament and position of males vis-à-vis females were not universal inevitabilities. Mead found among the Arapesh that males and females possessed similar temperaments in that both were rather passive, eager to please, compliant, and child-oriented. In contrast, she found the Mundugumor to be fierce, aggressive, highly sexed, exploitative, and not particularly child-centered. Once again, however, she found that males and females possessed a similar temperament. In her third group, the lake-dwelling Tchambuli, Mead found that the women were the entrepreneurs. They aggressively went and bartered at the marketplace, they did shrewd business, they were somewhat intrusive, and they admired and made comments about young men from a distance. She felt that males in this society were more passive and demure in their behavior. Much of their time was spent in frivolous body adornment or weaving and they would frequently walk down the path with a "mincing gait," hoping to catch the eye of an admiring woman. Mead concluded that temperament is obviously variable in the human situation; that females are not universally and inevitably passive, receptive, compliant, and child-oriented; nor are males masterful, aggressive, independent, and exploitative. Instead, she argued, as did Benedict, that what is normal for one society may not be normal for another; that a normal Tchambuli or Mundugumor woman would be quite out of place among the Arapesh. A normal Arapesh or Tchambuli man would be quite out of place among the Mundugumor. In addition, Mead argued that a woman's biology is not her destiny, that temperamentally her potentials are not different from those of a man.

During this period, in 1927, Bronislaw Malinowski published his work *Sex and Repression in Savage Society* (5). Malinowski did his fieldwork in the Trobriand Islands of Melanesia. He lived there for two years and observed that the family configuration in the Trobriands differed considerably from the family configuration in Western Europe. He found in the Trobriands that descent is traced through the female line rather than through the father. At birth, a boy becomes a member of his mother's clan. While the boy knows his biological father, he is most in awe of his mother's brother who is the main provider and disciplinarian of the boy's household. A boy's biological father provides for and exercises authority over his sister's household in a nearby village. In youth, the boy leaves his father's house, sometimes for long periods, to go to learn proper behavior from his maternal uncle. Malinowski observed that boys in Trobriand society seem to have no enmity whatsoever for their own fathers; in fact, they relate in a playful, relaxed way with them. On the other hand, they often resent the authority of their maternal uncles and at times evidence repressed hostility toward them. In addition, in this society there are no explicit taboos against mother-son incest, instead very clear regulations prohibit incest between brother and sister.

Once again, we have a noted anthropologist taking a position against the universalistic theoretical notions of Western psychiatry. In this case, Malinowski proposed that the Oedipus complex is purely a product of the family structure of the Victorian European household, where the biological father was an authoritarian individual and served as a realistic interferer with the close mother-son relationship. Father was thus naturally seen as a rival and a threat with whom the young boy had to come to terms. In the Trobriands, on the other hand, Malinowski pointed to a different kind of complex. Here the boy does not hate his father but his maternal uncle. Nor does he desire incest with his mother, since no taboos exist that prohibit such behavior. Instead he apparently desires incest with his sister, for which there exist abundant taboos. Malinowski went on to argue that perhaps each society has a characteristic complex in the same manner that Mead and Benedict argued that each society has its own particular temperament or ethos.

Today, many of these arguments seem to be cliché or even naïve. However, they did provide a healthy antithesis to the somewhat self-assured, complacent position of many analytic thinkers of that era. These observations from the field demanded more critical clinical examination, more enlightened theory, and undoubtedly served as forerunners of not only developments in ego psychology, but also the cultural relativist position of scholars such as Karen Horney.

Freudian psychology continued to inspire research in culture and personality despite these antithetical arguments. The idea that cultural institutions, such as curses, rituals, belief systems, folklore, art, and religion, may in part represent collective projected fears, wishes, and conflicts is a notion that has been very influential in psychocultural analysis. This idea was Freud's. In "The Future of an Illusion" (6), Freud studied the themes that constitute the core of religious phenomena and detected a correspondence between the methods men use to approach, communicate with, and control their deities and the experience they have had with their parents. The Judeo-Christian God was thus recognized as the projected image of Western man's stern, patriarchial father. Freud was on the brink of a new technique. For the first time, he described here the origin of what may be called a projective system, that is, a system for structuring the outer world and one's relation to it in accordance with a pattern laid down in an earlier childhood experience.

Abraham Kardiner, a psychoanalyst, Ralph Linton, an anthropologist, and others at Columbia proceeded to elaborate a rather simple schema demonstrating the relation between childhood events, personality, and subsequent fantasy systems.

Socialization Practices	→	Basic Personality	→	Projective Systems

The formula is obviously derived from what has been found to be true for the individual in analysis. Here, however, the formula is applied to the collective. In this case, the focus is not on an individual's childhood events and memories, but on group patterns of child rearing. The principle demonstrated here is that, especially in small, isolated, tradition-oriented societies, child-rearing practices will be more or less uniform from family to family. Consequently, most members of the society will develop core personality characteristics in common—"basic personality." Furthermore, there will be psychological needs, fears, and conflicts held commonly by the people and these will find expression not only in individual neurotic traits but in shared ritual and belief—"projective systems."

The link between child rearing and projective systems has been demonstrated through several studies using an extensive cross-cultural index (Human Relations Area Files) developed at Yale University (7–10). Each of these studies tends to support the general hypothesis that harsh parental treatment during infancy leads to the cultural belief that the spirit world is harsh and aggressive. Spiro and D'Andrade (7), using the Whiting and Child (8) "initial satisfaction of dependence" as a score for estimating the degree to which infants were indulged, found that societies judged to be relatively high on the above score tended to believe that the behavior of the gods was contingent upon the behavior of humans and that gods could be controlled by the performance of compulsive rituals. Such societies did not propitiate the gods. These authors argue that the adults' treatment of the gods is a reflection of an infant's relation to his parents. In other words, infants who are treated indulgently by their parents feel they can be equally successful in controlling the supernaturals when they grow up. Lambert, Triandis, and Wolf (9) used a score taken from Barry, Child, and Bacon (10) for estimating the relation between an infant and his caretakers, consisting of a judgment of the degree to which they treated him harshly or painfully. They found that societies in which infants were treated painfully believed in gods who were judged to be more aggressive than benevolent toward human beings. Again the gods seem to reflect the parental treatment of infants. Finally, Whiting (11), using still a different score for infant indulgence, reports a finding consistent with this hypothesis. The score in this study is also from Barry, Child, and Bacon (10) and is an overall judgment of the degree to which an infant is indulged by his caretakers. It was reported that societies high in the overall indulgence of infants tended not to fear ghosts at funerals. The assumption here is that funeral ghosts are, like the gods in the previous studies, a projection of the parental image.

Notice that the methods involved in studies are dependent on ethnographic descriptions of "child-rearing practices" and "projective systems," from which aspects of "basic personality" are inferred. This level of inference carries some uncertainty, as would the interpretation of a dream based on a carefully taken developmental history in an individual patient. In psychoanalysis such speculation might be useful in alerting the analyst to listen for confirmation or disconfirmation in the patient's free associations. Anthropologists have for the most part been limited in the past to collecting observable data on child rearing and projective systems. Rarely have studies included data on personality; and even more rarely have these descriptions of personality been based on the gathering of long-term, free-associative material. It should therefore not be too surprising that occasionally the inferences generated in such studies have subsequently proved unverifiable.

Wild analysis of projective systems earned psychoanalytic speculations and some skepticism from anthropologists. An example of a projective system which has been especially compelling and controversial is that involving surgical mutilations of a boy's penis. Often these rites are performed at puberty and may involve circumcision, superincision, and/or subincision. The nature of these rituals immediately conjures images of certain vicissitudes of the Oedipus complex.

Bruno Bettelheim published a book on this subject entitled *Symbolic Wounds* (12). In this work he argued that circumcision and especially subincision are not derivatives of castration at all, but represent identifications and wishes of the males to bleed and have a hole like a female— and to symbolically give birth to the emergent bodkin-glans. He cited the following Australian Aboriginal myth as demonstrating the equivalence between circumcision and menstruation.

> The originator of circumcision is described as a semihuman bird, one of the totemic ancestors. This bird once threw a boomerang, and as it returned, it circumcised the bird and entered the vulvas of *his* wives, cutting them internally so that they bled. This caused their monthly menstrual periods.

Bettelheim felt that this myth reflects the fact that Aboriginals consider menstruation to be a consequence of circumcision, and that, just as procreation in women cannot take place before they begin to menstruate, circumcision is a precondition for procreation in men.

Róheim (13), another psychoanalyst who was interested in these rites and who had the advantage of direct field experience with Aboriginals, had previously come to conclusions different from those of Bettelheim. Róheim investigated the details in ritual and myth of this projective system. He pointed out that until the rite, the boy is considered attached to mother and like a woman. Before the rite, the future father-in-law may have sexual relations with the boy "as if he were a woman." After the operation, the foreskin is preserved and then given back to the boy, who in turn gives it to his father-in-law in exchange for his wife. Here Róheim would agree with Bettelheim in equating the foreskin with the vagina. He believed, however, that the dynamic is oedipal—that the father is separating the son from the mother through the act of castration, at the same time initiating the boy into identification with manhood.

Anthropological research (11) using the cross-cultural correlation method previously mentioned (HRAF-Yale) has found the following relationships to hold in many societies around the world: exclusive mother-child residence and harsh initiation rites.

Exclusive mother-son residence with father essentially absent from the household during the developmental years of the boy is thought to generate either (1) a primary feminine identification which is both expressed and denied by the puberty rites (the Bettelheim hypothesis) and/or (2) a strong attachment to mother and competition with father with genital mutilation representing a counterphobic defense (the Freud-Róheim hypothesis).

Looking further for correlations that might shed additional understanding on these rites, Whiting and his co-workers found that circumcision can be statistically correlated with a pattern of social institutions and ecological constants. Cross-culturally, these rites have been found to occur statistically most frequently in the tropics; in societies with a prolonged post-partum sex taboo; where exclusive child-mother residence is common; and where women primarily work in small garden plots harvesting carbohydrate-rich foods and the diet is low in protein, occasionally resulting in clinical *kwashiorkor*. Such societies are most commonly patrilocal, and patrilineal, and practice polygamy. In addition, men often live together in a large communal dwelling. These authors point to a complex web of overdetermined or multiply determined behavior. The culture of societies existing over long periods of time in areas providing little protein food has evolved so as to adjust to these limitations. A developing child is assured of protein intake during crucial years of his early life by prolonged breastfeeding. This, in itself, inhibits ovulation for some time. However, such societies also practice a prolonged post-partum sex taboo which further limits fertility and ensures the child a longer stay at the breast. Furthermore, the prolonged sexual inavailability of the female, as well as the economic value of the female in farming fields, creates certain pressures on the male to accumulate more females—thus the practice of polygamy. In such a situation, it is more parsimonious to have a new bride live near her husband, hence patrilocality, and to have all children trace their descent through the male patrilineage. The prolonged exclusive child-mother residence is felt to create especially close bonds between the mother and the child which become problematic in later life. The female must ultimately leave her mother and move to the place of her husband. Similarly, the male child must leave his mother at a certain age and join the men's society. These traditions create many anxieties and conflicts in identity formation which are felt to be partially solved through the harsh rites of passage. Circumcision and other genital mutilations are seen in this context to represent a counterphobic defense against a fantasied all-powerful father and his group.

These studies are most enlightening in that they point out how integrally linked are fantasies and defenses (even ritualized defenses) with not only child-rearing patterns but also other elaborate complexities of social structure; and how all these traits may ultimately be in the service of biological adaptation. In this case, low availability of protein elicits a chain of cultural responses which include circumcision and subincision. Here culture may provide an additional dimension to phylogenesis as a complex determinant of these rituals.

Returning for a moment to the Kardiner formula relating child-rearing practices—basic personality—and projective systems, it is obvious that the above studies have emphasized the analysis of projective systems; they have analyzed child-rearing practices to a lesser degree; but direct information from the actual personalities to assist in interpreting these rituals is lacking. Responding to this lack of primary-informant data, John Cawte, a psychiatrist in Australia, collected a number of associations made by Aboriginals to questions regarding subincision rites (14). He asked:

1. Whether subincision is just a custom—Aboriginals replied, "It's the law. Every boy one day must have a *burra*."

2. Whether subincision is done for hygienic reasons—"With a *burra* the stream is wide and washes the penis out."

3. Whether subincision is used as an initiation—"It's the way to manhood . . . to go through it you must take rubbish and teasing . . . with pain . . . you get respect."

4. About contraception—"With a *burra*, you get more children, not less. And quicker. That's a fact . . . The width and spread helps. It doesn't flatten out inside the woman."

5. About simulation of women—"Sometimes we say, for a joke to certain friends, your *burra* is just like a *tjindi* . . . Young lovers compare

burra and *tjindi*, playing out in the bush. They look a little bit alike ...
Burra blood is not connected with women's blood in menstruation
though."

6. "*Burra* blood is easier to get than arm blood if you are in a
hurry. Sometimes it comes out too quick ... Sometimes it is hard to
get arm blood, and more sore afterwards. There is less pain when you
prick the *burra* ... The blood is no different, not more special or sacred
... Arm blood is better than *burra* blood for drinking during initiation ..."

7. "If you want to know about *Burra*—it's to be found in the
Dreaming not in your questions. It is explained in the stories. This
is from the Dreaming."

> The kangaroo on a journey met a little [marsupial] mouse,
> who knew nothing of drawing blood. They made a camp and
> the kangaroo said he'd show the mouse something he hadn't
> seen before—how to draw blood. The kangaroo sang some
> lovely tunes that the mouse hadn't heard before, and the mouse
> became very interested and excited. At last the kangaroo said,
> "Look away." Then he began to draw blood from his burra
> with a stick and pour it around the mouse's shoulders. The
> mouse was frightened but asked to learn the song and sing it
> while the kangaroo danced with his burra flashing up and down
> with the stick in it. The mouse asked the kangaroo to cut a
> burra for him, which the kangaroo did. You can still see the
> burra on the mouse; only a little thing, but you can see it.

Róheim (13) himself heard similar stories about subincision and
with his keen sense for detail reported that:

> All wildcat ancestors are supposed to have a double penis, and
> the subincised penis in the state of erection really looks some-
> what like a double penis. Among their Western neighbors with
> the kangaroo myths, the blood is derived from the subincised
> penis. Initiation rites are always performed in connection with
> kangaroo or euro ceremies.
>
> In the ritual the actors flicked their penes up and down,
> showing the fresh subincision wound. One of the performers
> pulls his penis violently and shakes it.
>
> He looks at it; it is not sufficiently erect; he is dissatisfied.
> He stabs the subincision wound to draw blood. Now they all
> twirl their penes around their fingers and when they are satisfied
> with the erection achieved, they hop backwards in a row, shout-
> ing "Pu, pu." Four men stand in a row pulling their penes

violently and making circular movements in front of the penis with the firestick. Blood runs down their legs. They flick the penis upward making a movement as if they were throwing something behind their backs, and run backwards like kangaroos.

Aboriginals imitate their totem animals—in dance, in body makeup, and song—particularly kangaroos. Cawte and his team were struck with the omnipresence of kangaroos and other marsupials in the stories about subincision, and decided to look and see if these animals indeed possess a subincision.

In 1704 Cowper had described that the male opossum possess a double or forked glans penis, and that many marsupials possess a grooved penis, and in general his descriptions corroborate the observations of the Walibiri Aborigines on the "subincision" of their totem animals (14). In Walibiri eyes, the animals do have a kind of *burra*. The Walibiri hypothesis about the relation between this anatomy and their own practice of subincision might be expressed:

1. The reasons we slit the penis lie in the dreaming and are explained in the stories.

2. Since we are kin with the animals and many of the animals slit the penis, this is one reason why it is an important thing for us to have a slit penis.

Freud once remarked that sometimes a cigar is just a cigar; in this case we too have a rather concrete equivalence. As interesting as the various hypotheses regarding the psychological meaning of genital initiation mutilations were, they were obviously inadequate and incomplete without more evidence from the fantasies and free associations of the Aboriginal. Cawte asked good questions, but may have obtained only surface material about the meanings of these rituals.

Anthropologists are increasingly becoming aware that psychoanalytic theory is predicated on using the psychoanalytic method. Good fieldwork is in many ways parallel to a good analysis. Much time and the gradual unfolding and reflecting of free associations *of the subject* is necessary before defenses begin to fall and deeper levels of the unconscious are realized. Thus, work in psychoanalysis and anthropology today focuses carefully on primary free-associative material from the native informant. The obvious symbolic meaning of certain projective systems can alert the fieldworker to certain psychological dynamics which must then eventually be verified through a long process of rapport, inquiry, and reduction of defensiveness.

Cross-cultural psychoanalytic investigation has moved closer to the informants in the field in finding answers to theoretical questions posed. Cultural psychiatry, as a broader field of inquiry, has moved in a similar manner to rely increasingly on good field methods to obtain accurate data. Such work involves considerable knowledge of the culture and of the people studied.

We have carefully selected the chapters of this volume to reflect the current emphasis on *clinical*, in-depth experience with patients of other cultures. Where theory is presented, it is based on years of study and experience with the subjects. Cultural psychiatry utilizes as many approaches to the understanding of human behavior and psychopathology as does the field of psychiatry itself. These various approaches are evident in this volume.

This chapter has attempted to review the changing relation between anthropology, psychoanalysis, and psychiatry. Cultural psychiatry has had its "ups-and-downs," but for the most part it has evolved into an increasingly vital, relevant aspect of psychiatry today.

REFERENCES

1. Freud, S. Totem and taboo. *Standard Edition of the Complete Psychological Works of Sigmund Freud,* Vol. XIII, ed. J. Strachey. London: Hogarth Press, 1913–1914.
2. Benedict, R. *Patterns of Culture.* New York: Mentor Books, 1959.
3. Mead, M. *Coming of Age in Samoa.* In: *From the South Seas.* New York: William Morrow, 1939.
4. Mead, M. *Sex and Temperament in Three Primitive Societies.* New York: Mentor Books, 1950.
5. Malinowski, B. *Sex and Repression in Savage Society.* London: Routledge & Kegan Paul, 1953.
6. Freud, S. The future of an illusion. *Standard Edition of the Complete Psychological Works of Sigmund Freud,* Vol. XXI, ed. J. Strachey. London: Hogarth Press, 1927–1931.
7. Spiro, M., and D'Andrade, R. A cross-cultural study of some supernatural beliefs. *Amer. Anthropol.,* 60: 456–66, 1958.
8. Whiting, J., and Child, I. *Child Training and Personality: A Cross-Cultural Study.* New Haven: Yale University Press, 1953.
9. Lambert, W., Triandes, L., and Wolf, M. Some correlates of beliefs in the malevolence and benevolence of supernatural beings: A cross-cultural study. *J. Abnorm. Soc. Psychol.,* 58: 162–68, 1959.
10. Barry, B., Child, I., and Bacon, M. Relation of child training to subsistence economy. *Amer. Anthropol.,* 61: 51–63, 1959.
11. Whiting, J. Socialization process and personality. In: *Psychological Anthropology,* ed. F. Hsu. Cambridge: Schenkman, 1961.

12. Bettelheim, B. *Symbolic Wounds*: *Puberty Rites and the Envious Male.* Glencoe, Ill.: Free Press, 1954.
13. Róheim, G. *Children of the Desert.* New York: Basic Books, 1974.
14. Cawte, J. *Medicine Is the Law.* Honolulu: University of Hawaii Press, 1974.

2

Psychodynamic Processes and Institutional Response: A New Rapprochement

WALTER GOLDSCHMIDT

BACKGROUND

Anthropology and the psychological disciplines have from the outset been closely associated. From the very birth of anthropology the influence of psychology has been apparent. Franz Boas was deeply influenced by Wilhelm Wundt and his understanding of culture always had a large psychological component.

Anthropology's involvement with psychiatry emerged with its adoption of some Freudian perceptions in the 1920's. Earlier, Alfred Kroeber endeavored to engage in psychotherapy—a little known and even less well-understood chapter in the life of that seminal member of the anthropological fraternity. The major thrust into psychological anthropology derived largely from Edward Sapir and Ruth Benedict. Indeed, Sapir (1) wrote a paper entitled "Why the Anthropologist Needs the Psychiatrist" published in the first issue of *Psychiatry*.

One of the early dialogues between anthropology and psychiatry was that between Malinowski (2) and the Freudian scholar Ernest Jones (3). Malinowski, using as always his data from the Trobriand Islanders, challenged the Freudian theory of the Oedipus complex. He argued that the psychological relationships characterized as oedipal derive not from the sexual basis Freud attributed them to, but rather from the more generic social relationships in the family constellation. Among the matrilineal Trobrianders, the father plays an avuncular role while the mother's brother plays the role we attribute to the fathers. Malinowski found that the relationship between the son and the mother's brother (who has no sexual access to his sister and indeed is forbidden to have social intercourse with her) contains the hostility Freud attributed to oedipal jealousies. This suggested to him that situational factors rather than sexuality are at the base of this dynamic element in individual psychology. Whether Malinowski was right—we all know that his analysis has been contested—is less important than the recognition that this controversy offers a paradigm for the developing relation between anthropology and psychiatry, and thus foreshadows matters to be discussed later.

An extensive investigation of psychological problems in cross-cultural perspective by what came to be known in anthropology as the "culture and personality" school followed these early ventures. The major pioneers of this activity were Margaret Mead, who was engaged in understanding the psychodynamics of child development from a cross-cultural perspective, Ralph Linton, who worked in close collaboration with Abram Kardiner, Clyde Kluckhohn, who collaborated with Murray and others at Harvard, Gregory Bateson whose work is too involved and too well known to require any elaboration here, A. I. Hallowell, who pioneered cross-cultural use of the Rorschach, and Geoffrey Gorer, who essayed psychoanalytic interpretations of Russian and American culture. Investigations of American Indian cultures from a psychodynamic viewpoint were engaged in in relation to Plains Indian culture, Pueblo cultures, and (by Erik Erikson) in northwestern California. The movement was almost entirely American, with the exception of Malinowski and Gorer.

The psychological and psychiatric involvement waned rapidly after World War II. Among the major reasons for this decline were, I believe, the following:

1. It was limited largely to Freudian perceptions of the dynamics of psychological aspects of behavior.

2. The reasoning was essentially circular in that it explained the dynamics of child rearing in terms of culture and culture in terms of the dynamics of child rearing; it therefore could not explain the *differences* between cultures, which is the essential task of anthropology.

3. It rarely examined one of the essential anthropological problems,

namely, the character of institutions as distinct from individual patterns of behavior.

4. It lacked any methodology by which there could be replication or verification.

There were situational reasons for this waning of interest as well. The expanding internationalism of the cold-war period drew anthropologists out of the country and toward more social, political, and economic problems. The early deaths of Sapir, Benedict, Linton, Kluckhohn, and Malinowski also decimated the ranks of the pioneers. Some, like Cora DuBois and A. I. Hallowell, turned away from these interests. For some reason, also, neither a special organization nor a special journal developed that might have given the movement coherence. Many anthropological editors were hostile to psychological material. Nevertheless, a legacy of interested and productive scholars, such as J. W. M. Whiting, Weston La Barre, Melford Spiro, and A. F. C. Wallace kept the spirit of this interest alive—although certainly not well.

Anthropology had a greater influence on psychiatry. The major conflicts between cultural anthropology and Freudian theory lay in the matter of instincts, in Freud's too facile establishment of general characteristics of the human psyche based on culture-bound observations, as expressed in the Malinowski-Jones controversy. The neo-Freudian movement in this country was a recognition of the force of culture in shaping the psychodynamics of human growth. Certainly those psychiatrists who have had the greatest public impact, those whose writings are part of the social philosophy of the day, were heavily influenced by anthropology. These include Karen Horney, Erikson (who worked among Indian cultures, as already noted, in close collaboration with anthropologists), Eric Fromm (who also has worked in alien cultures in collaboration with anthropologists), William Alanson White, and Judd Marmor. These diverse scholars, whatever the internal differences of their orientation, share a recognition of the essential cultural forces at work in the development of the individual and thus reject a good deal of Freudian orthodoxy.

The long "latency period" in the relation between psychiatry and anthropology seems to be coming to a close. Evidence of this new rapprochement between the two fields is indicated by the appearance of new journals in both psychology and anthropology. It is true that the *Journal of Cross-Cultural Psychology* is more psychological than psychiatric, but this is part of the shift in orientation. The journal *Ethos*, edited jointly by myself and Professor Douglass Price-Williams, a psychologist with broad cross-cultural experience and anthropological interests, is perhaps more catholic in its orientation. I might add, parenthetically, that we developed this journal in conscious recognition of the need for an institutional home for those interested in the relation between the cultural-social and the psychological elements in human behavior.[1] This symposium, held in conjunction with the American Psychiatric Association, is further evidence of a similar sentiment stemming from the other side.

THE PSYCHOLOGICAL ELEMENT IN INSTITUTIONAL BEHAVIOR

It is my conviction that the anthropologist must involve himself with psychological understandings in order to explain that which is his province to explain: the nature of institutionalized behavior and the variation in such behavior. During the post-war years, anthropology has been dominated by sociological reasoning, the major elements of which are the necessity of explaining social phenomena in sociological terms and the obverse of this, the strict taboo on "reductionism." The essential vacuity of this thesis is now generally beginning to emerge. In the remainder of this paper, I shall illustrate that we cannot understand institutions without a recognition of their psychological dynamics, as these operate within the context of a set of economic circumstances, i.e., the ecology.

Let me start with some consideration of that hardy perennial of anthropological discourse: kinship. A major thrust of kinship studies has been the demonstration that kinship systems are arbitrary, that the genealogical chart is irrelevant to an understanding of kinship, and that the sooner we remove it from our systemics the quicker we will be able to understand the phenomenon.

This is arrant nonsense. Of course tribal peoples do not concern themselves with the transmission of DNA, but the genetic model supplies the social model. Children are still conceived through an act of copulation; the mother lactates and in perhaps 99 percent of all instances in every society (except certain middle- and upper-class sectors of advanced communities) she nurses the infant and has major responsibility for his early nurturance. In perhaps only 90 percent of the instances, the presumptive genitor has the second primary role in infant nurturance. These primary relationships, together with the relationship derived from close sharing of these nurturant adults (i.e., siblings), form the basis of every known kinship system, which is built by compounding them. (It is not insignificant that the terms for these primary relationships are universally made up of contrasting sets of easily formed, often reduplicative syllables—baby talk. Mama, papa, baba, dada, kaka appear over and over again, though often with their referents reversed. Nor is it insignificant that George Murdock's paper [4] describing this has been so little valued—even by Murdock himself.)

The important point is that it is not the *genetics* of biological relationships but the *sentiments* of domestic relationships that make a kinship system a kinship system. The pattern of attachment, to use John Bowlby's (5) term, is the focal element in the systematic use of kinship by tribal societies in organizing their social life—and which we ourselves have not abandoned. If we are to understand kinship as a phenomenon, we must examine the dynamics inherent in the early infantile experience. For it is in the psychology of the domestic scene that the sentiments are established by which social cohesion is attained.

This matter leads me to another consideration. René Spitz (6) discusses the coenesthetic sensibility of the infant (and the mother), what Freud called "primary process thought." He suggests that ritual practices evoke these elements in tribal societies, referring to the process as *regression*. Aside from the negative implications of this word choice (which apparently reflects his attitude), the matter is of central importance. Indeed, I believe that it is quite impossible to understand the functions, let alone the forms, of ritual behavior unless we recognize that they evoke sentiments laid down in infancy, particularly in the experience of the mother-infant dyad. Every politician knows this when he evokes home and mother in his Independence Day speeches, but anthropologists have been slow to appreciate this lesson. Rather than speak of regression to the infantile level, we should recognize that rituals characteristically *mobilize the sentiments laid down in infancy for the performance of socially relevant actions.*

A third example of the dynamics of psychological development for the formation of institutions will be taken from my work among the Sebei of Uganda (7). Like so many societies that require strong masculine bonds, the Sebei engage in initiations of classic proportions. The focal element of this rite, which takes place in early manhood, is circumcision, but it also includes temporary extrusion from the community in a period of isolation, with the familiar theme of death and rebirth. These rituals are designed to perform two functions: to transform youths into men (i.e., to serve as rites of passage), and to bond together into formal age-sets the young men who must work in concert to care for the herds, to protect them from raiders and to raid those of their neighbors (i.e., to serve as a rite of intensification).

To understand the form of these rituals, as Whiting and his associates (8) have shown, it is necessary to recognize the need to transform youths from family dependency to independent, acting-out militants. At the same time, it is essential that they be bonded into a cohesive force—hence group rather than solitary initiations. When Sebei culture began to change from pastoralism to farming, a process that began before Europeans entered the area, the usefulness of age-sets was undermined. Indeed, the formation of groups of men bonded together as military units can be counterproductive. As a result of this ecologic change, the age-set system rapidly lost its functions, and new community-based institutional patterns had to be developed to meet the new needs. The decline of pastoralism and the sedentation of the people created localized tensions which inspired new legal organizations and altered ritual patterns. Thus, for instance, a ritual designed to alleviate tensions between kindred (particularly affinals) was altered to relieve tensions between neighbors.

Among the Sebei, women are also initiated with a "circumcision" involving a labiedectomy, which leads me to another observation of the psychological relevance of institutionalized behavior—this time a coping mechanism. One of the worst things that can befall an initiate is to "cry the knife," as the Sebei refer to any failure to complete the operation in perfect stoic control. One girl refused to let the operation be completed, to the distress of her kindred and the bemusement of all others. Ultimately she was held down and the operation performed. When I called on her a week or so later, expecting to find her in deep depression and self-hatred, she was to my surprise in no such condition. While she still had to suffer the social disabilities for her failure, the culture provided her with an institutionalized ego defense. She knew who had made her cry the knife. It was a man whose advances she had rebuffed some months earlier and who had performed witchcraft. Seen in such a light, witchcraft beliefs do not seem to have quite the unmitigated evil that we are wont to ascribe to them.

This matter of witchcraft leads to one further example of the need to understand psychological processes if we are to understand institutional variation. My study of the Sebei was part of a larger study involving four tribes, each of which had the internal variation between farming and pastoralism described for the Sebei. We postulated that there would be a higher incidence of witchcraft concern among farmers, because farmers must suppress their feelings since they must live indefinitely in close proximity to their neighbors. We found that the pastoralists generally were more open in their expression of affect and that they did display less concern with witchcraft—in three of the four instances. Insofar as three out of four can be said to constitute cor-

roboration, this exemplifies the relation between psychodynamics, ecological circumstances, and the character of institutions.

The validity of this conclusion rests on understanding the situation
in the fourth, the recalcitrant tribe, the Kamba. Among the Kamba of
Kenya, witchcraft accusations were widespread in both areas, but were
clearly more intense in the pastoral sector. It is relevant that the
pastoral Kamba are the most gynophobic people I have ever read about;
they hate and distrust their wives with institutionalized fervor. It is
considered very bad form for the man to give sexual satisfaction to his
wife. The result, deriving no doubt from affect hunger on both sides
of the bed, is that there is a great deal of clandestine extramarital sexual
activity. The men who do not give their wives satisfaction seek and
satisfy other men's wives and beat their wives for being involved with
other men. In the farming sector, sexual dalliance and intersexual hatred
is nowhere near as pervasive.

An understanding of why the pastoral Kamba behave in this way
tells us something about the relation between psychodynamics and
institutions. The pastoral Kamba are not so much pastoralists as *frustrated* pastoralists. The youths are socialized to a pastoral kind of
existence in a series of rituals, the last of which is much more hazardous
and demanding than the Sebei's circumcision—which is certainly hazardous and demanding enough. Socialized to this masculine activity
through informal and formal techniques, youths emerge from their
initiation unable to fulfill the roles to which their indoctrination adapts
them. Presumably, these Kamba had in the past the animal-herding,
militaristic, male-bonded life for which these initiations prepared them.
But nowadays they have only a few miserable cattle; governmental
controls and Masai power prevent them from expanding such an
economy over the grasslands. Instead, they (or rather their wives)
scratch out a hard and niggardly living by farming dry patches of
land. This is an activity that produces no wealth and little satisfaction,
as it does in the true farming sector. Instead, young initiates form
dancing groups, and together with girls and unmarried women spend
long hours in social dancing which displays a peculiar combination of
sexuality and close-order drill. Needless to say, this is accompanied
by a good deal of extramarital sexual activity. Many men hang on to
this period of irresponsible sexuality and quasi-military activity until
they become so old that younger men begin to tease them; ultimately,
they seek wives and establish households.

In this pattern of socialization, the men turn their frustration against
their hard-working wives who symbolize for them their failure to
engage in the activity they were taught to believe is ego gratifying.

It is not surprising, given this social background, that sexual dalliance continues after marriage. Nor is it surprising that this leads to a great deal of witchcraft—particularly witchcraft between husbands and wives. It is a situation that Ruth Benedict (9) called "discontinuities in cultural conditioning," an example of the malfunctioning of institutionalized behavior that is maladapted because it relates to a no longer viable situation.

IMPLICATIONS FOR PSYCHIATRIC PRACTICE

If institutions serve psychological functions, and if, as some of my illustrations indicate, they may fail to serve psychiatric functions, then an understanding of social institutions is important to the psychiatrist. In this closing section, I shall illustrate this point with a specific example from recent American history.

Let us consider the discontent of the late sixties. Without discounting the importance of the disastrous wars in Southeast Asia and the trauma of the Kennedy assassinations, I think the discontent of the period— a discontent by no means abated, but now more diversely institutionalized—sprang from the absence of what I would call avuncular substitutes. We know from tribal society how often the uncle (normally the mother's brother) plays a role in short-circuiting the generation gap. Having a representative of the older generation with whom one has no structured hostility (whether Freudian or Malinowskian), is an important intergenerational communicative device. The uncle in our society is supposed to play this role, but our highly mobile, scattered society leaves many youths without this important, though largely unrecognized, role relationship. The preacher (outmoded) and the "shrink" (overpriced) often serve as surrogates. The professor has classically been another such surrogate.

The counterculture movement began in the universities, in particular, in those universities known for their academic excellence, as best represented by Berkeley. While the obvious function of the university is the transmission of knowledge and its perfection, its secondary and latent function is to provide a period of transition for youth, comparable to the initiations among the Sebei and Kamba. But as we all know, as a byproduct of the efflorescence of academia, professors became increasingly involved in their academic activities at the expense of their teaching and counseling functions—in what has been called "the leisure of the theory class." As a result, the students, particularly in the bigger universities, were not served with this avuncular role. When they could not communicate with those whose counsel they needed, they turned on their professors and tried "to shut down the universities." Whenever a population acts in a self-destructive manner, it is useful to examine what institutional failures have developed as unanticipated consequences of other changes.

SUMMARY

I have tried to illustrate what I think is the new relation between the social and the psychological disciplines. The examples deal with institutionalized rather than idiosyncratic forms of behavior. From the anthropological standpoint, I am more interested in the way psychological and psychodynamic elements help to shape institutional forms. From the psychiatric standpoint, it is an understanding of institutions as they shape individuals, and particularly malfunctioning institutions as they fail to shape individuals into functionally useful members of the community, that is primary. I believe this to be the essential element in the interdependence of the social and the psychological disciplines.

[1]The leaders in the development of *Ethos* were Spiro, Theodore Schwartz (who has worked in close collaboration with Mead) at the University of California, San Diego, my own former students Robert B. Edgerton and John Kennedy of the Neuropsychiatric Institute at UCLA, and George DeVos and Herbert Philips, at Berkeley. We early coopted Mead and Robert LeVine and we have conscientiously sought more involvement from psychiatrists and psychologists (as our masthead indicates), but have been less successful in getting either manuscripts or subscriptions from outside anthropology than we had hoped.

REFERENCES

1. Sapir, Edward. Why the Cultural Anthropologist Needs the Psychiatrist. *Selected Writings of Edward Sapir* (D. Mandelbaum, ed.), Berkeley and Los Angeles: University of California Press, 1949, pp. 569–577. (First published in *Psychiatry*, Vol. I, 1938.)
2. Malinowski, Bronislaw. Psychoanalysis and Anthropology, in *Sex, Culture and Myth*, New York: Harcourt, Brace and World, 1962, pp. 114–116. (First published in *Nature*, Nov. 3, 1923).

3. Jones, Ernest. Mother-Right and the Sexual Ignorance of Savages, *International Journal of Psycho-analysis*, VI, Part 2, 1925, pp. 109–130.

4. Murdock, George P. Cross-Language Parallels in Parental Kin Terms, *Culture and Society*, Pittsburgh: University of Pittsburgh Press, 1965, pp. 325–330. (First published in *Anthropological Linguistics*, Vol. I, No. 9, 1959.)

5. Bowlby, John. *Attachment and Loss*, Volume I, *Attachment*. New York: Basic Books, 1969.

6. Spitz, R. *The First Year of Life*. New York: International Universities Press, 1965.

7. Goldschmidt, W. *Culture and Behavior of the Sebei*. Berkeley and Los Angeles: University of California Press, 1976.

8. Whiting, John W.M., Richard P. Kluckhohn and Albert S. Anthony, The Function of Male Initiation Ceremonies at Puberty. *Readings in Social Psychology* (Maccoby, Newcomb and Hartley, eds.) New York: H. Holt, 1958, pp. 359–370.

9. Benedict, Ruth. Continuities and Discontinuities in Cultural Conditioning. *Psychiatry*, Vol. I, pp. 161–167, 1938.

3

Anthropological and Cross-Cultural Themes in Mental Health

ARMANDO R. FAVAZZA
MARY OMAN

The term "behavioral scientist" includes professionals in many fields. A psychiatrist is a behavioral scientist who, at least theoretically, must synthesize pertinent data from the areas of biology, psychology, sociology, and anthropology. In practical terms, the psychiatrist must attempt to comprehend daily those biological, psychological, and sociocultural forces that enhance or impede a patient's mental health and functioning. In medical school the training of all physicians focuses primarily on biological functioning. During psychiatric residency training the student adds information about psychological functioning to his repertoire and also learns about selected sociological concepts. The introduction of sociological input during the past two decades has been great and is due, in large part, to the development of the community health movement. Studies, such as that by Hollingshead and Redlich (1), brilliantly added the sociological dimension to psychiatric understanding.

The cultural dimension, or what can be more broadly termed the anthropological dimension, has not yet been fully appreciated by psychiatrists. To be sure, there have been great collaborative efforts, such as those by Sullivan and Sapir, the Leightons and Kluckhohn, Kardiner and DuBois—but these are relatively few. Transcultural psychiatry is a relatively small subspecialty, and it is the one area of psychiatry that has attempted to incorporate anthropological data. The first book devoted to transcultural psychiatry was written by Kiev (2) in 1972.

Our interest in the psychiatric-anthropological interface matured with the realization that psychiatrists and anthropologists share many common interests. We believe that the development of an interface science should be based on a knowledge of themes common to the interfacing disciplines. We began by preparing articles on three themes (the Oedipus complex, national character, and feral man), attempting to synthesize the psychiatric and anthropological perspectives for each theme. An inordinate amount of time was devoted to developing a bibliography on each topic and we considered the idea of compiling a comprehensive bibliography of anthropological and cross-cultural themes in the mental health literature. An NIMH computer search was not very helpful since the computers were not programmed to fit our needs. Driver's *The Sociology and Anthropology of Mental Illness* (3) was helpful, but it, too, was not exactly what we had in mind. Driver's book lists 5,910 titles of articles and books published between 1956–1968. The titles were selected by searching seven major bibliographic sources. A substantial number of the articles did not seem relevant to our project. We also found that, by relying on bibliographic sources rather than going to the journals themselves, Driver did not have access to some articles which were clearly anthropological. Examples of such articles are R. Firth's "Suicide and Risk-Taking in Tikopia Society" (4) and E. Preble's "Social and Cultural Factors Related to Narcotic Use among Puerto Ricans in New York City" (5).

We then decided to develop a bibliography by going to the journals themselves and reviewing every article. After some consultation we settled on 68 psychiatric and psychological journals for review. We realize that the list is arbitrary, but we believe we have included all the major English-language journals in the field. All the large-circulation journals, such as the *American Journal of Psychiatry, British Journal of Psychiatry, Journal of Social Psychology,* and *Child Development* were included, as were smaller-circulation journals, such as *American Imago, Journal of the History of Behavioral Sciences,* and the *Journal of Operational Psychiatry.* Four journals devoted to marriage and family studies were included. In general, then, our list is fairly comprehensive.

The starting date for our review was 1925. At that time, some psychiatrists and anthropologists were bitterly embroiled over the interpretation of Malinowski's Trobriand data as it affected the concept of the universality of the Oedipus complex. We felt that the perspective of half a century would make our bibliography more useful. Our data span the period 1925–1974.

SELECTION OF ARTICLES

Because of the almost limitless topical orientation of anthropology the selection of articles with anthropological and cross-cultural relevance was problematic. We selected those articles we felt most anthropologists would identify and accept as "anthropological" in subject matter and/or approach. We searched for key concepts, such as cultural system, tribe, native, ethnology, and race, as well as articles that focused on non-Western cultures and groups. Articles dealing with subcultures in peasant and industrial society and urban life were selected as they reflected anthropology's increased recent concern with complex society. Most of the articles did not possess a truly anthropological method-ological and theoretical orientation. Our bibliography thus reflects material that could be a valuable research tool rather than being a compilation of anthropological orientations per se.

The following are examples of articles that are clearly anthropo-logically oriented:

Seligman, C.G. Temperament, conflict and psychosis in a stone-age population. *Brit. J. Med. Psychol.*, 9:187–202, 1929.

Henry, J. Anthropology and psychosomatics. *Psychosom. Med.*, 11:216–222, 1949.

Turnbull, C.M. Some observations regarding the experience and behavior of the BaMbuti pygmies. *Amer. J. Pschol.*, 74:304–308, 1961.

Abernethy, V. Dominance and sexual behavior: A hypothesis. *Amer. J. Psychiat.*, 131:813–816, 1974.

We used our best judgment in selecting articles and in borderline cases we reviewed an article's bibliography. If clear-cut anthropological sources were listed, we tended to include the article. Because of the difficulty in trying to differentiate clearly between anthropological and sociological themes, we adopted a liberal policy of inclusion, as we felt it would make the bibliography a more helpful document.

Many of the cross-cultural articles do not possess a true anthropo-logical orientation. They do, however, provide data amenable to cultural and social research and which add to the information included in the

Human Relations Area Files. Most of these articles do not consider cultural influences as primary to the investigation, and in only a few is the material synthesized.

MAJOR FIELDS OF ANTHROPOLOGY

Our bibliography contains 3,624 articles. Dividing these into the four major fields of anthropology, we find that 3,169 can be classified under the broad heading of Cultural Anthropology; 297 fall under Physical Anthropology; 180 under Linguistics; and 10 under Archeology.

The following are examples of typical articles for each major category:

Cultural Anthropology

Jones, E. Mother-right and the sexual ignorance of savages. *Internat. J. Psycho-Anal.*, 6:109–130, 1925.

Lambo, T. Psychotherapy in Africa. *Psychother. Psychosom.*, 24:311–326, 1974.

Physical Anthropology

Clegg, J.L. The association of physique and mental condition. *J. Ment. Sci.*, 81:297–316, 1935.

Gluck, J.P. and Sackett, G.P. Frustration and self-aggression in social isolate Rhesus monkeys. *J. Abnorm. Psychol.*, 93:331–334, 1974.

Linguistics

Wolfe, D.L.L. The role of generalization in language. *Brit. J. Psychol.*, 24:434–444, 1934.

Miller, P.M. A note on sex differences on the semantic differential. *Brit. J. Soc. Clin. Psychol.*, 13:33–36, 1974.

Archaeology

Kohen, M. The Venus of Willendorf. *Amer. Imago*, 3:49–60, 1946.

Ward, T.H.G. An experiment on serial reproduction with special reference to the changes in design of early coin types. *Brit. J. Psychol.*, 39:142–147, 1949.

CULTURAL AREAS

Many articles deal with specific populations and with geographically delimitable culture areas. When broken down by culture area, we found articles dealing with Asia numbered 555, followed by American sub-cultures (418), Africa (317), Europe (309), Native America (250), Mideast (209), Latin and South America (191), and Oceania and Australia (154).

As well as general articles in the Asia category, there are articles dealing with the following areas and peoples: Afghanistan, Ainu, Arakan, Atayal, Batak, Borneo, Burgher, Burma, Cantonese, Ceylon Tamil, Cha-morro, China, Communist China, Hong Kong, Iban, India, Indonesia, Japan, Korea, Korea South, Laos, Malaysia, Meo, Mongols, Moslem, Murut, Nuristani, Okinawa, Pakistan, Pakistan East, Pakistan West, Philippines, Saipan, Sarawak, Semang, Senoi, Singapore, Sri Lanka, Sumatra, Tagalog, Taiwan, Thailand, Tibet, Tungus, Vietnam. Articles on India (191) formed the largest group, followed by articles on Japan and Japanese, China and Chinese, and the Philippines. Only two articles, surprisingly, deal with Vietnam.

Included in the *American Subcultures* category are articles on the following: Amish, Appalachia, Chinese-American, Doukhobor, Danish-American, Filipino-American, French-American, French-Canadian, Ger-man-American, Greek-American, Haole, Hutterite, Hawaiian, Hawaiian-Filipino, Hawaiian-Japanese, Hungarian-American, Irish-American, Issei, Italian-American, Italian-Canadian, Japanese-American, Jewish-American, Korean-American, Mennonite, Mexican-American, Negro, Nissei, Nor-wegian-American, Okinawan-American, Oriental-American, Polish-Amer-ican, Samoan-American, Scandinavian-American, Slovak-American, Swed-ish-American, Swiss-American. The majority of the articles deal with Negroes with special attention to the subheadings of cognition, family, identity, intelligence, mental disorder, and personality.

Included in the *Africa* category are general articles as well as articles on the following areas and peoples: Agni, Afrikaners, Akan, Amhara, Ashanti, Bacongo, Bakitara, BaMbuti, Bushmen, Bantu, Banyan-kole, Bashi, Bassa, Belgian Congo, Bena Bena, Chagga, Congo, Dogon, East Africa, Egypt, Egypt (ancient), Ethiopia, Ewe, Fan, Fang, French Guinea, Ga, Gabonese, Ganda, Ghana, Gold Coast, Gusii, Hausa, Hutu, Ibibio, Ibo, Ibusa, Kafa, Kamba, Kasangati, Katangese, Kenya, Kikuyu, Kipsigi, Kpelle, Lesu, Liberia, Logoli, Logos, Luo, Lusaka, Malawi, Mano, Mashona, Mauritius, Morocco, Ngoni, Nigeria, Nsenga, Nupe, Nyanja, Nyasaland, Onitshas, Rhodesia, Rwanda, Serer, Senegal, Sierra Leone, Soli, Somali, Sousou, South Africa, Sudan, Swazi, Tanzania, Temne, Tiv, Togoland, Tunisia, Uganda, Ugandan Asians, Wabena, Wapogoro, West Africa, Wolof, Xhosa, Yao, Yoruba, Zambia, Zulu. Ethiopia, Ghana, Kenya, Nigeria, South Africa, Uganda, and Zambia are heavily repre-sented areas. The Bantu and Yoruba are the two tribes about which the most articles have been written.

Included in the *Europe* category are general articles as well as articles on the following areas and peoples: Austria, Balkans, Belgium, Bulgaria, Croatia, Czechoslovakia, Denmark, Dinaric Alps, France, Finland, Germany, Great Britain, Greece, Hungary, Ireland, Italy, Komi Republic, Kvaen, Lapp, Norway, Netherlands, Poland, Scandinavia, Scotland, Sicily, Slovenian, Sweden, Switzerland, United Soviet Socialist Republic, Wales, Yugoslavia, Zadruga, Zyrians. Great Britain and Germany are the two areas most often represented. Articles on national character form an interesting subgroup in this category, especially those dealing with the supposed "paranoid" trends in German culture.

The *Native American* category includes general articles on North American Indians, as well as articles on the following North and South American native groups: Aleut, Andean Indian, Apache, Athabaskan, Blackfoot, Bororo, Camba, Canadian Indian, Carrier, Cheyenne, Chilcotin, Chippewa, Coast Salish, Coconuco, Cree, Dakota Indian, Digueno, Eskimo, Forest Potawatomi, Guatemalan Indians, Hopi, Indian-Metis, Iroquois, Kaska, Mapuches, Maya, Menomini, Mistassini Cree, Mohave, Navaho, Nez Perce, North American Indians, North Pacific Coast Indians, Ojibwa, Osage, Paiute, Papago, Pawnee, Peruvian Indian, Pilaga, Pima, Plateau Indian, Plains Indian, Pomo, Quekchi, Quiche, Salteaux, Saskatchewan Indians, Seminole, Sioux, Tarahumara, Teton Dakota, Toltec, Tsimshian, Ute, Wintu, Yakima, Yuma, Yurok, Zuni, Zia. The groups about which the most articles were written are the Apache, the Eskimo, and the Navaho.

Included in the *Mideast* category are general articles, as well as articles on the following areas and peoples: Arab, Arab-Gulf states, Bedouin, French-Arab, Iran, Iraq, Israel, Jew: Iranian, Jew: Iraqui, Jew: Yemenite, Lebanon, Moslem, Palestinian, Saudi Arabia, Shirazi, Turkey. Many of the articles (81) stem from Israel, and the majority deal with studies of the kibbutz.

The category *Latin and South America* includes general articles, as well as articles on the following areas and groups: Argentina, Bahamas, Barbados, Black Carib, Bolivia, Brazil, British Honduras, British Guiana, British West Indies, Caribbean, Chile, Colombia, Costa Rica, Cuba, Dominican Republic, Grand Cayman, Grenada, Guatemala, Guyana, Haiti, Jamaica, Ladino, Menjala, Meso America, Mestizo, Mexico, Mocheros, Montserrat, Netherlands West Indies, Peru, Puerto Rico, St. Thomas, Tobago, Trinidad, Uruguay, Yucatan, Zapotec, Zinacanteco. Brazil, Mexico, and Puerto Rico are the areas about which the most has been written.

Our last category, *Australia and Oceania*, includes general articles as well as articles on the following areas and peoples: Alorese, Arapesh,

Australia, Bali, Dobu, Fijian, Fore, Guam, Gururumba, Ifaluk, Maori, Marquesas, Melanesia, Mundugamor, Normanby Island, New Britain, New Guinea, New Ireland, New Zealand, Papua, Polynesia, Ponape, Pukapuka Atoll, Samoa, Tahiti, Tikopia, Tolai, Tonga, Trobriands. This category also includes general articles on Australian aborigines, as well as articles on the following aboriginal groups: Aranda, Arnhemland, Arunta, Bamyili, Hooker Creek, Kimberly, Lardil, Walbiri, Warburton Ranges, Western Desert, Yolngu, Yowera.

SPECIFIC THEMES

In addition to examining culture areas and groups, we divided the articles into 24 specific anthropological cross-cultural themes. These themes are General Culture, Psychiatry and Personality; Child Rearing and Socialization; Ritual, Religion, and Mythology; Folklore and Dreams; Native Medicine and Psychotherapy; Psychotherapy: General; Acculturation and Immigration; Aggression; Testing Performance and Technique; Cross-Cultural Research; Culture, Mental Illness and Mental Health; Incest, Freudian Concepts, and Oedipus Complex; Sexuality, Sex Roles and Sex Behavior; Values, Roles, and Attitudes; Drug and Alcohol Use; Race and Racism; Constitution and Physical Types; Nonhuman Primates; Ethology; General Physical Anthropology; Social Class, Economy, and Politics; Family, Marriage, and Kinship; Language and Communication; Cognition.

General Culture, Psychiatry and Personality is the most heterogeneous category and contains 560 references. The following are examples of articles:

Sapir, E. The emergence of the concept of personality in a study of culture. *J. Soc. Psychol.*, 5:408–415, 1934.

Opler, M.K. Cultural perspectives in mental health research. *Amer. J. Orthopsychiat.*, 24:51–59, 1955.

Rodreigues, A. and Comrey, A.L. Personality structure in Brazil and the United States. *J. Soc. Psychol.*, 92:19–26, 1974.

Leff, J.P. Culture and the differentiation of emotional states. *Brit. J. Psychiat.*, 123:299–306, 1973.

Child Rearing and Socialization contains 148 references, most of which were written after 1950. Examples include:

Havighurst, R.J. Child development in relation to community social structure. *Child Devel.*, 17:85–89, 1946.

Tulkin, S.R. and Liederman, P.H. Infancy in a cultural context:

Caudill's contribution to comparative child development. *J. Nerv. Ment. Dis.*, 157:320–322, 1973.

Madsden, M.C. and Kagan, S. Mother-directed achievement of children in two cultures. *J. Cross-Cult. Psychol.*, 4:221–228, 1973.

Ryback, D. Child rearing and child care among the Sino-Thai population of Bangkok. *J. Soc. Psychol.*, 92:307–308, 1974.

Ritual, Religion, and Mythology provided 108 references. Examples include:

Cheney, C.O. The psychology of mythology. *Psychiat. Quart.*, 1:198–209, 1927.

Schnier, J. The Tibetan Lamaist ritual: Chod. *Internat. J. Psycho-Anal.*, 38; 402–407, 1957.

Ozturk, O. Ritual circumcision and castration anxiety. *Psychiatry*, 36:49–60, 1973.

Chaudhuri, A.K.R. A psychoanalytic study of the Hindu mother goddess (Kali) concept. *Amer. Imago*, 13:123–146, 1956.

Folklore and Dreams contributed only 43 references. Examples include:

Karno, M. and Edgerton, R.B. Some folk beliefs about mental illness: A reconsideration. *Internat. J. Soc. Psychiat.*, 20:292–296, 1974.

Lee, S.G. Social influences in Zulu dreaming. *J. Soc. Psychol.*, 47:265–283, 1958.

Native Medicine and Psychotherapy provided 78 references, most of which were written after 1960. Examples include:

Freedman, L.Z. and Ferguson, V.M. The question of "painless childbirth" in primitive cultures. *Amer. J. Orthopsychiat.*, 20:363–372, 1950.

Jilek, W.G. and Todd, N. Witchdoctors succeed where doctors fail. Psychotherapy among Coast Salish Indians. *Can. Psychiat. Assn. J.*, 19:351–356, 1974.

Wintrob, R.M. The influence of others: Witchcraft and rootwork as explanations of behavior disturbances. *J. Nerv. Ment. Dis.*, 156:318–326, 1973.

Lewis, T.H. An Indian healer's preventive medicine procedure. *Hosp. Commun. Psychiat.*, 25:94–95, 1974.

There are 124 articles under *Psychotherapy: General*. Most were written after 1955, and they point out the influence of culture on the practice of psychotherapy. Examples include:

Henry, J. The formal social structure of a psychiatric hospital. *Psychiatry*, 17:139–151, 1954.

Mayo, J.A. The significance of sociocultural variables in the psychiatric treatment of black outpatients. *Compr. Psychiat.*, 15:471–482, 1974.

Wittkower, E.D. and Warnes, H. Cultural aspects of psychotherapy. *Amer. J. Psychother.*, 28:566–573, 1974.

Young, B. and Kinzie, J.D. Psychiatric consultation to a Filipino community in Hawaii. *Amer. J. Psychiat.*, 131:563–566, 1974.

Acculturation and Immigration provided 144 references. Examples include:

Hallowell, A.K. Values, acculturation and mental health. *Amer. J. Orthopsychiat.*, 20:732–743, 1950.

Danziger, K. The acculturation of Italian girls in Canada. *Internat. J. Psychol.*, 9:129–137, 1974.

Seguin, C.A. Migration and psychosomatic disadaptation. *Psychosom. Med.*, 18:404–409, 1956.

Stromberg, J., Peyman, H., and Dowd, J.E. Migration and health: Adaptation experiences of Iranian migrants to the city of Teheran. *Soc. Sci. Med.*, 8:309–323, 1974.

The category *Aggression* contains only 83 references, a surprisingly small number for such an important category. Examples include:

Westermeyer, J. Assassination in Laos. *Arch. Gen. Psychiat.*, 28:740–743, 1973.

Gluck, J.P. and Sackett, G.P. Frustration and self-aggression in social isolate Rhesus monkeys. *J. Abnorm. Psychol.*, 83:331–334, 1974.

Meyer-Bahlburg, H., Boon, D., Sharma, A., and Edwards, J. Aggressiveness and testosterone measures in man. *Psychosom. Med.*, 36:269–274, 1974.

Worchel, S. Societal restrictiveness and the presence of outlets for the release of aggression. *J. Cross-Cult. Psychol.*, 5:109–123, 1974.

The category *Testing Performance and Technique* contains 404 references which deal with a great number of primarily psychological instruments. Examples include:

David, K.H. Cross-cultural use of the Porteus Maze. *J. Soc. Psychol.*, 92:11–18, 1974.

Deregowski, J.B. Effects of symmetry upon reproduction of Kohs-type figures: An African study. *Brit. J. Psychol.*, 65: 93–102, 1974.

Honess, T. and Kline, P. The use of the EPI and the JEPI with a student population in Uganda. *Brit. J. Soc. Clin. Psychol.*, 13:96–98, 1974.

Sachs, D.A. The WISC and the Mescalero Apache. *J. Soc. Psychol.*, 92:303–304, 1974.

Cross-Cultural Research provided 479 references, most of which were written after 1955. Examples include:

Prothro, E.T. Arab-American differences in the judgment of written messages. *J. Soc. Psychol.*, 42:3–12, 1955.

Adams, E.M. and Osgood, C.E. A cross-cultural study of the affective meanings of color. *J. Cross-Cult. Psychol.*, 4:135–156, 1973.

Barraclough, B.M. Differences between national suicide rates. *Brit. J. Psychiat.*, 122:95–96, 1973.

Wagner, D.A. The development of short-term and incidental memory. A cross-cultural study. *Child Devel.*, 45: 389–396, 1974.

Culture, Mental Illness and Mental Health, a category of special interest to the clinician, provided 375 references. Examples include:

Foulks, E.F. and Katz, S. The mental health of Alaskan natives. *Acta Psychiat. Scand.*, 49:91–96, 1973.

Gobeil, O. El Susto: A descriptive analysis. *Internat. J. Soc. Psychiat.*, 19:38–43, 1973.

Beiser, M., Buri, W.A., Collomb, H., and Ravel, J.L. Pobough Lang in Senegal. *Soc. Psychiat.*, 9:123–129, 1974.

Burke, A.W. Socio-cultural aspects of attempted suicide among women in Trinidad and Tobago. *Brit. J. Psychiat.*, 125:374–377, 1974.

Burton-Bradley, B.G. Social change and psychosomatic response in Papua, New Guinea. *Psychother. Psychosom.*, 23:229–239, 1974.

Fabrega, H. Problems implicit in the cultural and social study of depression. *Psychosom. Med.*, 36:377–398, 1974.

Incest, Freudian Concepts, and Oedipus Complex were grouped into one category which yielded 54 references. Examples include:

Devereux, G. The social and cultural implications of incest

among the Mohave Indians. *Psychoanal. Quart.*, 8:510–533, 1939.

Schwartzman, J. The individual, incest and exogamy. *Psychiatry*, 37:171–180, 1974.

Favazza, A. Oedipus interruptus: A psychiatric-anthropological interface. *J. Oper. Psychiat.*, 5:37–51, 1974.

Vesky-Warner, L. An Irish legend as proof of Freud's theory of joint parracide. *Internat. J. Psycho-Anal.*, 38:117–120, 1957.

Sexuality, Sex Roles and Sex Behavior contributed 116 references. Examples include:

Benedict, R. Sex in primitive society. *Amer. J. Orthopsychiat.*, 9:570–573, 1939.

Hobart, C.W. Sexual permissiveness in young English and French Canadians. *J. Marr. Family*, 34:292–304, 1972.

Green, R. and Fuller, M. Family doll play and female identity in preadolescent males. *Amer. J. Orthopsychiat.*, 43:123–127, 1973.

Whiting, B. and Edward, C.P. A cross-cultural analysis of sex differences in the behavior of children aged three through eleven. *J. Soc. Psychol.*, 91:171–188, 1973.

Values, Roles, and Attitudes contains 325 references. Most of these articles do not deal with values and attitudes as broad theoretical concepts but rather as specific measures of cultural differences and personality configurations. Examples include:

McIntire, W.G., Ness, G.D., and Dreyer, A.S. A cross-cultural comparison of adolescent perception of parental roles. *J. Marr. Family*, 34:735–740, 1972.

Radke, M. and Trager, H. Children's perceptions of social roles of Negroes and whites. *J. Psychol.*, 29:3–34, 1950.

Gardiner, H.W. Human figure drawings as indicators of value development among Thai children. *J. Cross-Cult. Psychol.*, 5:124–130, 1974.

Sutcliffe, C.R. The effects of differential exposure to modernization on the value orientations of Palestinians. *J. Soc. Psychol.*, 93:173–180, 1974.

The category *Drug and Alcohol Use* contributed 101 references. Examples include:

Horton, D. The functions of alcohol in primitive societies: A cross-cultural study. *Q. J. Stud. Alcohol*, 4:199–320, 1943.

Bales, R.F. Cultural differences in rates of alcoholism. *Q. J. Stud. Alcohol*, 6:480–499, 1946.

Ewing, J.A., Rouse, B.A., and Pellizzari, E.D. Alcohol sensitivity and ethnic background. *Amer. J. Psychiat.*, 131:206–210, 1974.

Westermeyer, J.A. Opium smoking in Laos: A survey of 40 addicts. *Amer. J. Psychiat.*, 131:165–170, 1974.

Race and Racism contains 87 references and they are fairly evenly distributed over time from 1925–1974. Examples include:

Katz, D. and Braly, K.W. Racial prejudice and social stereotypes. *J. Abnorm. Soc. Psychol.*, 30:175–198, 1935.

Adinarayan, S.P. A study of racial attitudes in India. *J. Soc. Psychol.*, 45:211–216, 1957.

Orpen, C. and Tsapogas, G. Racial prejudice and authoritarianism. A test in white South Africa. *Psychol. Rep.*, 30:441–442, 1972.

Lamont, J. and Tyler, C. Racial differences in rate of depression. *J. Clin. Psychol.*, 29:428–432, 1973.

Constitution and Physical Types contributed only 54 references. This category contains items which are more of historical than practical interest to psychiatrists. Examples include:

Barahal, H.S. Constitutional factors in psychotic male homosexuals. *Psychiat. Quart.*, 13:391–400, 1939.

Parnell, R.W. The Rees-Eysenck body index of individual somatotypes. *J. Ment. Sci.*, 103:209–213, 1957.

Lerner, R.M. and Korn, S.J. The development of body-build stereotypes in males. *Child Devel.*, 43:908–920, 1972.

Polednak, A.P. Body build of paranoid and non-paranoid schizophrenic males. *Brit. J. Psychiat.*, 119:191–192, 1971.

The *Nonhuman Primate* category contributed 84 references. Much significant work in this area stems from researchers at the University of Wisconsin and Stanford University. Examples include:

Baldwin, J.D. and Baldwin, J.I. The dynamics of interpersonal spacing in monkeys and man. *Amer. J. Orthopsychiat.*, 44:790–806, 1974.

Reite, M., Kaufman, I.C., Pauley, J.D. and Stynes, A.S. Depression in infant monkeys: Physiological correlates. *Psychosom. Med.*, 36:363–367, 1974.

McKinney, W.T. Primate social isolation. *Arch. Gen. Psychiat.*, 31:422–426, 1974.

Van Lawick-Goodall, J. The behavior of chimpanzees in their natural habitat. *Amer. J. Psychiat.*, 130:1–12, 1973.

The category *Ethology* contains 68 references. Examples include:

Edney, J.J. Human territoriality. *Psychol. Bull.*, 81: 959–975, 1974.

White, K.G., Jukhasz, J.B., and Wilson, P.J. Is man no more than this? Evaluative bias in interspecies comparison. *J. Hist. Behav. Sci.*, 9:203–212, 1973.

Shenken, L.I. An application of ethology to aspects of human behavior. *Brit. J. Med. Psychol.*, 46:123–134, 1973.

Jones, I.H. Stereotyped aggression in a group of Western Desert aborigines. *Brit. J. Med. Psychol.*, 44:259–265, 1971.

General Physical Anthropology provided 89 references and is a heterogeneous category. Examples include:

Montagu, A. The physical anthropology of the American Negro. *Psychiatry*, 7:31–44, 1944.

Henton, C.L. A comparative study of the onset of menarche among Negro and white children. *J. Psychol.*, 46:65–74, 1958.

Kiritz, A. and Moos, R.H. Physiological effects of social environments. *Psychosom. Med.*, 36:96–114, 1974.

Kuglemass, S., Lieblich, I., and Ben-Shakhar, G. Information detection through differential GSR's in Bedouins of the Israeli desert. *J. Cross-Cult. Psychol.*, 4:481–492, 1973.

Social Class, Economy, and Politics, another heterogeneous category, provided 72 references, many of which have a sociological theme. Examples include:

Brody, E.B. Psychiatric implications of industrialization and rapid social change. *J. Nerv. Ment. Dis.*, 156:300–305, 1973.

Munroe, R.L., Munroe, R.H., and Daniels, R.E. Relation of subsistence economy to conformity in three East African societies. *J. Soc. Psychol.*, 89:149–150, 1973.

Barron, F. and Young, H.B. Personal values and political affiliation within Italy. *J. Cross-Cult. Psychol.*, 1:444–468, 1970.

Michael, S.I. A social class dependent factor in questionnaire research. *J. Psychiat. Res.*, 10:73–82, 1973.

The category *Family, Marriage and Kinship* provided 322 references, with a sharp increase noted after 1960. While there undoubtedly has been an increase in attention to family studies, our figures may be an artifact of our inclusion of four specialty journals (*Journal of Marriage and the Family, Family Coordinator, Marriage and Family Living,* and *Family Process*). Examples include:

Koomen, W. A note on the authoritarian German family. *J. Marr. Family,* 36:634–636, 1974.

Smith, H.E. The Thai family: Nuclear or extended. *J. Marr. Family,* 35:136–141, 1973.

Veevers, J. The social meanings of parenthood. *Psychiatry,* 36: 291–310, 1973.

Kinzie, D., Sushama, P.C., and Lee, M. Cross-cultural family therapy—A Malaysian experience. *Fam. Process,* 11:59–68, 1972.

The *Language and Communication* category includes 183 references. Examples include:

Tuckman, J. and Ziegler, R. Language usage and social maturity as related to suicide notes. *J. Soc. Psychol.,* 68:139–141, 1966.

Johnson, F.A., Marsella, A.J., and Johnson, C.L. Social and psychological aspects of verbal behavior in Japanese-Americans. *Amer. J. Psychiat.,* 131:580–583, 1974.

Scherer, S.E. Proxemic behavior of primary school children as a function of their socioeconomic class and subculture. *J. Pers. Soc. Psychol.,* 29:800–805, 1974.

Weinstein, E.A. Symbolization and the Sapir-Whorf hypothesis. *Contemp. Psychoanal.,* 9:133–135, 1973.

Cognition, our last category, provided 173 articles, of which 120 were published since 1965. Examples include:

Stewart, V.M. A cross-cultural test of the "carpentered world" hypothesis using the Ames distorted room illusion. *Internat. J. Psychol.,* 9:79–89, 1974.

Youniss, J. and Dean, A. Judgment and imaging aspects of operations: A Piagetian study with Korean and Costa Rican children. *Child Devel.,* 45:1020, 1031, 1974.

Greenfield, P.M. Comparing dimensional categorization in natural and artificial concepts: A developmental study among the Zinacantecos of Mexico. *J. Soc. Psychol.,* 93:157–171, 1974.

Ramirez, M. and Price-Williams, D.R. Cognitive styles of children of three ethnic groups in the United States. *J. Cross-Cult. Psychol.,* 5:212–219, 1974.

THE FUTURE

Obviously the range in quality of the articles is quite great when one considers all 3,624 references. We have made no attempt to classify quality. That task belongs to future workers.

We would not have devoted so much time and energy to our effort had we not strongly believed that anthropological insights are potentially significant for psychiatry, and vice versa. We do not foresee any major "breakthrough," but rather hope for a gradual and continued sharing of information. In 1943 Gregory Zilboorg (6) noted, "Sociology and anthropology are increasingly intertwined with psychiatry." Thirty-three years later we note that psychiatrists make daily use of sociological information. Indeed, physicians in general are being exposed to sociologists in medical school, often in "behavioral science" or "human ecology" courses. Anthropology as a major behavioral science has not yet made a major impact on physicians in general, or on psychiatrists in particular. As our work shows, authors in mental health journals have certainly shown an interest in themes also of interest to anthropologists. We hope our work will prove to be a modest step forward in bringing psychiatry and anthropology closer together (7).

REFERENCES

1. Hollingshead, A., and Redlich, F. *Social Class and Mental Illness*. New York: Wiley, 1958.
2. Kiev, A. *Transcultural Psychiatry*. New York: Free Press, 1972.
3. Driver. . *The Sociology and Anthropology of Mental Illness*. Amherst: University of Massachusetts Press, 1972.
4. Firth, R. Suicide and risk-taking in Tikopia society. *Psychiatry*, 24: 1–17, 1961.
5. Preble, E. Social and cultural factors related to narcotic use among Puerto Ricans in New York City. *Internat. J. Addictions*, 1: 30–41, 1966.
6. Zilboorg, G. Psychiatry as a social science. *Amer. J. Psychiat.* 99: 585–588, 1944.
7. Favazza, A., and Oman, M. *Anthropological and Cross-Cultural Themes in Mental Health*. Columbia: University of Missouri Press, 1977.

4

A Gap Between Psychiatry and Underprivileged Groups

ARI KIEV

The most psychologically vulnerable minority groups in America are reservation Indians and northern ghetto dwellers, and yet only a negligible percentage receive appropriate care from the nation's 18,000 predominantly white, middle-class psychiatrists.

Can psychiatry, basically geared to middle-class values, prove meaningful to the ghetto dweller? Can the rural or urban slum dweller establish meaningful communication with the psychiatric profession in contexts other than impersonal state hospitals? Certainly the disadvantaged minorities experience much the same response from "the system" as other lower socioeconomic groups, with a disproportionate number being diagnosed as schizophrenic, and hospitalized in public facilities. The chain of events including police intervention, court certification, and state hospitalization occurs with much less frequency in middle-class or affluent patients with the same clinical problems.

What accounts for the obvious communication gap which still prevails between psychiatrists and minority-group members? Is this an economic problem or are other factors at work?

To understand the problem it is useful to first consider the nature of the vulnerability fostered by ghetto life. The lack of family supports and adequate models for identification, particularly among Indians on reservations and blacks in northern ghettos, reduces the chances for the development of good reality-testing ability, motivation for achievement, and cognitive skills for setting and reaching personal goals. This sociocultural dynamic process occurs with greater frequency in these groups and has differential effects on individuals depending on age of exposure to stress, age of deprivation, and the availability of supports. Yet certain attitudes occur with great frequency even among those without psychiatric problems. Uncertainty about opportunities creates confusion, pressure, and a sense of inadequacy among many, while increased dependence on others fosters low self-esteem and habits of compromise, which perpetuate a vicious circle of continued dependency.

Low self-esteem leads to a defensive denial of inner feelings of "weaknesses" and reliance on maintaining a false "image." Fear of discovery increases defensiveness and diverts energy from the development of coping skills, assertiveness, and increased self-mastery. The recurrent specter of unemployment further discourages efforts to utilize free time for personal growth. Unless the needs for housing, nutrition, and physical health are met, it is difficult to concentrate on self-development.

The culture of poverty complicates reservation and ghetto life not only by discouraging participation in the larger culture, but also by not providing meaningful traditions or satisfactory interpersonal relationships in the ghetto itself. Anomie and alienation flourish. Chronic apathy and negativism influence responses to illness. Attitudes toward seeking help often contain elements of hostility and dependency, which are notoriously difficult to cope with in any group of patients, irrespective of culture. A general lack of knowledge and familiarity with the medical care system and a distrust of hospitals in general are special features encountered with disadvantaged patients.

The ghetto dweller with attitudes developed in a rural agrarian environment and/or the culture of poverty often lacks the skills and comprehension for managing in the social system. The perception of limited opportunities to adapt to particular environments more than reality factors themselves often contributes to individual failure to adapt successfully to ghetto stresses. In addition to the objective stresses encountered by everyone in the educational and occupational spheres, the ghetto dweller must contend with discriminatory practices, and perhaps most important, a range of attitudes fostered in the ghetto itself that reinforce a negative self-image and a rather hopeless, futile expectation of self. The absence of constructive channels for aggression leads to the diversion of suppressed aggression into self-destructive channels. The high rate of suicide, homicide, alcoholism, and drug abuse among young men in northern ghettos and on Indian reservations attests to this underlying motivational pattern.

The greater the internal discomfort experienced, the more the individual experiences an urge to obliterate feelings of helplessness and hopelessness. Lack of cognitive appreciation of other options and lack of adaptive skills also make it difficult to cope with stress.

The culture of poverty thus fosters anomie and alienation from the larger society. Unsupported by traditions or family ties, cramped into impoverished and crowded quarters, lacking intellectual stimulation and encouragement of his human potential, the ghetto dweller often lacks the motivation to seek psychiatric help to improve his life. Confusion, conflict, contradictory desires, frustration, suspiciousness, competitiveness, and envy emerge when aspirations collide with reality.

Noncommitment and withdrawal become critical defense mechanisms in the face of reality, but they bring with them a negative self-image, a pessimism about the future, and minimal expectations about achievement for oneself or one's children. Feelings of inferiority inhibit involvement in psychotherapy, which emphasizes individual responsibility, and discourage psychiatrists who are accustomed to working with patients better equipped to implement the insights gained in psychotherapy. While a certain amount of stimulation and interaction with others promotes good mental health, excessive stimulation, as in crowded ghettos, produces negative effects by reinforcing dependency and reducing both autonomy and the value placed on such traits as perseverance and hard work, which facilitate adjustment in urban settings.

The street becomes an escape and a setting for socializing. Street heroes display their affluence and become role models for all who want to share in the material side of the American dream without following conventional routes of hard work and the postponement of gratification. The pressure to conform also operates on the street, making success through conventional educational and occupational channels anathema to many young people fearful of outstripping their peers. Ghetto dwellers' problems relate to police brutality, lack of jobs, bad housing, poor education, inadequate recreation facilities, biased justice, inadequate federal programs, and discriminatory credit practices. We know the handicaps of a history of slavery, exploitation, segregation, rural-urban migration, poverty, maternal deprivation, and unstable or weak family experiences. We know also of the Indian's loss of traditional culture and identity, and the dependency fostered by reservation life. Similarly, we grasp how the Chicanos have suffered from a conflict between traditional agrarian values and those of Anglo society. These varied experiences contribute to behavioral problems of low frustration tolerance, proneness to violence, problems in masculine identification, and antisocial behavior, all of which occur with great frequency in these population groups and are notoriously difficult to treat with the present tools of modern psychiatry.

Patients with behavior disorders lack the necessary tolerance of frustration and control of impulsivity to enable them to build a sustained relationship with a psychiatrist—the cornerstone of psychotherapy. And as yet, there are insufficient psychopharmaceuticals for managing such patients. The traditional psychotherapeutic emphasis on responsibility and autonomy often conflicts with the hostile and dependent attitudes of patients with behavior disorders. While psychotropic medications are useful in the management of symptomatic states, psychotherapeutic objectives and the techniques employed are constrained by the patient's capacity to initiate action and assume personal responsibility.

The general lack of techniques for treating many of the behavior disorders, coupled with the fallacy that these conditions are characteristic of the disadvantaged (erroneously assigning to the group as a whole the characteristics of individual patients) and the failure (from lack of contact and study) to differentiate between normal behavioral styles among the disadvantaged and behavioral disorders that accentuate these styles, has no doubt contributed to some of the disinclination of psychiatrists to take on such patients.

While behavior disorders are difficult to treat, neuroses and psychoses, which are fundamentally symptomatic conditions rather than behavioral disorders, can be treated successfully with medicine independently of the sociocultural origins of the patient. Symptoms of depression or schizophrenia are quite similar from culture to culture, the variation being in the patients' mental preoccupations which relate to culturally defined causative factors, stresses, and concerns.

The culture of poverty would appear to contribute to a greater incidence of illnesses characterized by behavioral disorders, such as psychopathy, alcoholism, and drug addiction, all of which tend to be less responsive to conventional psychiatric treatments, irrespective of the individual's background.

The tendency to associate the manifestations of certain syndromes to ethnicity or social class may often lead to an accentuation of the importance assigned to elements of these syndromes that appear in association with other syndromes, amenable to conventional treatment. So, the ghetto dweller's risk of getting inappropriate treatment is greater than that of white, middle-class patients, simply because of the "ecological fallacy" of attributing group characteristics to individual group members.

Reality factors invariably intrude in the treatment process and at times confuse both patient and therapist. Ultimately, however much the environment contributed to the patient's problems or prevented him from realizing his aspirations or implementing the insights gained in treatment, the psychotherapeutic task is a psychological one that differentiates between the patient and the environment.

The psychiatrist cannot change the patient's environment and indeed is likely to try to assist the patient to accept the world in existential terms. But this is precisely where the prospects for improved communication between the disadvantaged groups and middle-class psychiatrists have the greatest potential for positive interaction. For ultimately the psychological solutions most beneficial to the slum dwellers relate to the basic philosophical premises of psychiatry with its emphasis on autonomy, self-reliance, and personal responsibility. Most schools of psychiatry, the Black Muslims, and other self-help groups hold that the patient loses strength to the extent that he focuses energy on blaming the social system for his problems and seeks to find ways to redress his grievances. Rather, a genuine sense of identity and personal power ultimately derives from focusing attention on inner resources, the development of self-reliance and self-discipline, and the achievement of personal goals. By regaining inner confidence and freedom from concerns of acceptance by the larger social system or the ghetto subculture, which, too, can inhibit personal growth by demanding conformity, the individual becomes free. It is of interest to note that much of the leadership of the black movement supporting this emphasis on self-reliance comes from southern ministers with strong restrictions who have traditionally stressed self-reliance.

To achieve this self-disciplined state of mind, which harnesses the energy within the individual, requires an enormous amount of faith and a willingness to let go of conventional symbols of status and security, to withdraw from the torments challenging masculinity, and to accept one's lot in the belief that one must begin with one's own resources to truly overcome.

At times, this orientation, which strives to activate the patient's resources, does not fit the disadvantaged who cannot implement strategies learned in treatment because of political and economic impotence. An emphasis on autonomy and self-actualization may, for example, conflict with the high value placed on group solidarity and conformity in the culture of poverty. It may also appear to promise more than the individual can realize, given the limitations of the system.

The advent of goal-oriented crisis-intervention techniques using rapid-acting psychopharmaceuticals for symptom relief and psychotherapeutic sessions focused on pragmatic life strategies is increasingly proving relevant to assisting less privileged groups whose psychiatric problems are compounded from social and psychological issues. The disadvantaged present various challenges to those interested in developing rational strategies for assisting people in different sociocultural contexts. My own experience has relevance here. Recognizing the barriers to communication, I first began to function as a consultant, reducing my own anxiety about working with unfamiliar groups, establishing my own credibility, and at the same time, multiplying my own efforts by working with the leaders in specific programs. My own experience suggests that my functioning as a catalyst and educator proved useful in the development of residential programs run by ex-addicts; it has been possible to establish a position of acceptance in a ghetto community. Once having done this, it becomes relatively easy to establish working relationships with disadvantaged patients from the ghetto subculture. Ultimately, it is discomfort and a general lack of familiarity with the disadvantaged groups that keep most psychiatrists from dealing with them.

5

Transcultural Attitudes Toward Antisocial Behavior: Perceived Strategies for Social Control

JAMES M. A. WEISS
MARGARET E. PERRY

Antisocial and criminal behaviors are complex sociopsychiatric phenomena associated with highly charged affect. While there is general agreement that violent behaviors transgressing sociolegal norms are often symptomatic of underlying social and emotional dysfunction, those who deal with these phenomena on a professional level—psychiatrists, police, and court officers, for example—are clearly influenced consciously or unconsciously by cultural attitudes (1–3). Labeling theory, a major new direction in crime research developed during the 1960's, supports a focus on social control processes and social reaction to deviance (4). Törnudd, for example, suggests that searchers for the causes of crime should concentrate on the decisive part played by society and social values both in defining the nature of criminal behavior and in deciding how to deal with offenders (5).

Methodology for this series of projects was devised by Dr. Weiss while he was Visiting Professor at the Institute of Criminology, Cambridge University (England), 1968–69. Research associates and assistants who worked on the investigations include: Carol E. R. Bohmer, Gerald R. Chase, James N. Hogrebe, Camille P. Ressler, James A. Roller, Rodney W. Wall, and Jenny A. Weiss.

In this view, deviant behaviors essentially reflect the obverse of the norms and values of the larger community, which defines the rules by which certain behaviors come to be viewed as aberrant. Yet these public norms, values, and attitudes are generally implicit and have seldom been studied qualitatively. Törnudd indicates that such value judgments have become more diffuse as society has become more complex, which explains to some degree the often contradictory effects of social control efforts. Because, however, systems of criminal justice and programs of prevention, disposition, treatment, and rehabilitation cannot exist for long in the face of widespread public antagonism, and because either gradual or radical changes in public programs may influence, or be influenced by, public attitudes in various cultures, it becomes vital to understand how, in fact, the public feels about criminal events, the persons who precipitated them, and possible strategies for control.

Some investigations of this nature have already been undertaken. Mäkelä (6) in Finland, Hogarth (7) in Canada, Bohmer (8) and Watson and Sterling (9) in the United States have all investigated attitudes of members of the law enforcement and judicial systems toward crime and criminals. All found considerable variance among such subjects, but Hogarth's study indicates that magistrates' attitudes are the most important single factor in predicting their sentencing behavior, substantially more so than the factual makeup of the actual criminal cases. Hogarth found that the major portion of the variance in such attitudes could be related to three factors: the magistrates' perceived conflict between the needs of offenders and social constraints, the influence on the magistrates of other persons and external opinions, and a generalized bias against members of "outgroups."

Questions then arise as to how such variances are distributed among the general population, how antisocial behavior in general and the social reaction to it are determined by group values, and how different cultures may differ in this respect. Since Murdock (10) found that the only categorical, universal taboo (if any) in man's history appears to be mother-son incest, there is strong logical support for the argument that all other taboos (i.e., definitions of behavior as "antisocial"), as well as prescriptions for dealing with the violators of such taboos, must arise from the psychosocial development of individual human beings within groups and from group interactions. The variety of newer theories relevant to the etiology of delinquency and deviance (including some forms of mental illness), as reviewed by McCartney (4), implies an equally large variety of strategies for control of such behavior. "Labeling" perspective includes an insistence that antisocial or criminal attributes are not inherent properties of certain acts, but are rather the consequence of societal reaction to certain acts. Obviously then, it becomes of substantial importance that psychiatrists and others in the helping professions, who are becoming increasingly involved in evaluation, adjudication, and disposition processes directed toward transgressors of sociolegal norms, as well as in consultation concerning the development of social control strategies, be aware of the nature, quality, and distribution of such societal reactions to deviance.

For these reasons, the authors and several colleagues have developed a series of ongoing projects concerned with public attitudes toward crime and antisocial behavior in various cultures and subcultures. In the first two studies (11, 12), it was demonstrated that people in urban areas throughout much of the world are most concerned about crimes of violence (especially homicide) and theft, as well as exploitation and public dishonesty. Other kinds of "antisocial" behavior (including other kinds of life-threatening behavior) are apparently seen as important "crimes" by only relatively small groups of the public. Significant differences among respondents in defining the most serious crimes related primarily to geographic location, rather than to other demographic or educational variables. The present study attempts to delineate the variance in such public attitudes as they relate specifically to perceived strategies for social control of "antisocial" and criminal behaviors.

METHOD

Most studies of public opinion about any problem involve quantitative rather than qualitative sampling. However, by using Thompson's (13) schema for the measurement of *qualitative* attributes, Stephenson devoloped formal models (14–18) for the study of public opinion regarding complex problems, which are examined only superficially or not at all in current large-sample opinion-survey techniques that are solely quantitative. With such models one can compare and contrast attributes in different cultural settings, test the invariance of the factors, interpret consensus statements, and determine genuine segments of opinion about controversial matters in depth, in aspects hitherto untouched by mensuration.

For our series of studies, a modification of the Stephenson factorial design was devised to obtain a balanced sample of empirically derived, representative opinions by utilizing small-sampling techniques. This design allowed a stratified, quasi-balanced, factorial sampling of 30 to 35 subjects in each of eight large cities scattered throughout the world. The sampling technique provides for classes by age, sex, socioeconomic status, and degree of expertise and/or involvement to be represented in each city.[1]

Age groups were categorized as young (under 30 years of age), middle-aged (30 to 59 years old), and old (60 years old or over). Socio-economic class was determined by our modification of the Hollingshead-Redlich indices (19) in which only factors of education and occupation, which might be comparable internationally, were used. In essence, "upper class" was comprised primarily of executives, proprietors and managers of large or medium-sized concerns, major professionals (such as doctors, lawyers, or engineers), and lesser professionals (such as teachers, social workers, or pharmacists). In addition, administrative personnel of large concerns, owners of smaller independent businesses, and semiprofessionals (such as photographers, draftsment, some nurses at higher administrative levels) were generally classified "upper class" if they had attended college or university, and "middle class" otherwise. Other middle-class persons included owners of small businesses, clerical and sales workers, technicians, and skilled workers. The category "lower class" was comprised generally of semiskilled workers and unskilled workers, day laborers, and the chronically unemployed.

As to degree of involvement, "experts" were defined as those who had some substantial degree of authority, information, and knowledge in the subject, usually those with a considerable amount of special training and/or experience in some aspect of criminology. The "involved" or "special interest" category included persons who had some personal or occupational involvement with crime or criminals, or whose spouse,

---

[1]Stephenson (14–16) has demonstrated empirically that a random sampling of even 30 subjects in each geographic replication is adequate for making statistically significant comparisons, provided several persons in each "category of interest" are represented therein. Such sampling is "not by cell, but only to insure a representation of the segment." A complete balance is not necessary because of subsequent adjustment in the statistical analysis. For this study, interviewers generally selected 15 ± 5 subjects of each sex and 10 ± 4 subjects in each other demographic category segment, at each geographic location. The advantage in using this sampling technique is that interviewers are not forced to search for the difficult or impossible case, such as a lower-class female under 30 years of age who is also an expert, or to fill all 54 cells (2 sexes x 3 age groups x 3 socioeconomic classes x 3 degrees of involvement, at each location). As Stephenson (16) says, "By taking a few probings in different parts of the body public, each for no more than a set of forty persons, one [can] test the invariance of the factors and can make estimates as to the sizes of the important segments . . . enough for most pragmatic purposes. . ." (p. 287).

parent, child, or sibling was so involved, but who were clearly *not* experts. "The "uninformed, uninvolved" category included those subjects who had never had any relevant special education or training or formal occupational experience, or any personal involvement with crime or criminals.

Other requirements were that all subjects be at least 14 years or older, native-born in the country in which interviewed, have lived (and also have worked, if working) for 10 years or more in the city in which interviewed, and be able to communicate reasonably well (through an interpreter if required). All subjects in any particular city were also selected from the major racial or ethnic group predominant in that metropolitan area.

Each subject was interviewed and asked partially open-ended questions such as: "In your opinion, what are the five worst crimes anyone can commit?" "What are the best ways to deal with criminals? (Or crime?)" If the subject's answer included less than five discrete statements of opinion in each respect, or was unclear, he or she was asked to amplify. From the 258 respondents in the eight cities in this study (Athens, Bombay, Dublin, Istanbul, London, Paris, St. Louis, and Tokyo), a universe of 2,603 statements of opinion were derived.

These statements were then subjected to content analysis and categorized into various subsets (including those discussed here) relevant to the attributes of the various responses (whether or not the opinions implied confidence, prescribed action, were judgmental or distorted, or involved affect) and also into 15 empirically derived subsets of specific content, utilizing a balanced block design in both cases. A single statement could be categorized, of course, in more than one content subset— for example, the response "Murderers deserve to be executed" would be listed as traditional, moralistic, and punitive (concern for abstract justice).[2]

The data were then examined using an analysis of variance approximation. The response scores (numbers in each content category) were coded as the dependent variables and the demographic category classes (such as location, age, or sex) as the independent variables. Differences among the dependent variables were further investigated using the

---

[2]Content analysis and categorization were performed by both authors jointly after a "blind" comparison of 100 randomly selected statements indicated 98 percent congruence. For the smaller number of subsequent cases where such congruence was not immediate, agreement was usually reached after brief discussion. In 11 instances, agreement could not be reached and these 11 statements were discarded.

parameters in the statistical model. For example, the mean response score in each content category for each different location was computed after adjustment for all other independent variables (e.g., age, sex) was accounted for. *P* values of .05 or less were deemed to indicate statistically significant differences, and *p* values of .50 or more were deemed to indicate high probability of agreement among the various demographic subgroups.

This technique allows only for inference about general trends; comparison between demographic groups, however, can provide quite exact information by indicating the "proportion of responses" above or below the adjusted mean score of any demographic category class on any content category cell or subset.

RESULTS

The first noteworthy fact about the results was the rather high level of agreement in many response attributes among subjects in the eight very different cities, although the commonality of attitude *content* was by no means as consistent as in the same subjects' responses to the first major interview topic—the most serious crimes. Nevertheless, there was substantial agreement ($p > .50$) among various demographic subgroups in 46 out of 130 possible rating categories of "what to do about crime."

The great majority of respondents (98.4 percent) gave confident recommendations, i.e., statements asserted with conviction and (except for 3.1 percent) prescribing some definite course of action, policy, or direction. A clear majority (65.5 percent) endorsed a problem-solving approach indicating or implying some way of dealing with crime in an organized, step-by-step manner, and this was the most highly endorsed type of response in every location.

At this point, the commonality of attitudes diverged into two major subpatterns. A somewhat larger group of respondents (36.1 percent) endorsed *only* those content categories that could be subsumed under what might be called the traditional-moralistic orientation, in which crime seems to be regarded as "sin" and the way to deal with it primarily involves punishment. A somewhat smaller proportion of respondents (27.1 percent) endorsed only responses that could be subsumed under what might be called the public health model, in which crime seems to be regarded as "social illness" and the way to deal with it primarily involves general social programs to prevent or reduce crime, directly or indirectly, as well as treatment, rehabilitation, and/or re-education processes. A small group of subjects (8.1 percent) endorsed only responses emphasizing a need for more information or research, misapplication of selected information, a concern solely for humaneness, or entirely idiosyncratic concerns. For the remainder (28.7 percent), there were internal contradictions within the several responses of the same subject, so that in one opinion he or she might endorse capital punishment and in the next emphasize a need for more extensive treatment and rehabilitation programs (see Table 1). Even in this latter group, however, respondents endorsed more traditional-moralistic opinions, since 82.6 percent of *all responses* supported this orientation, while only 61.6 percent of all responses supported the public health orientation. This 4 to 3 ratio (of traditional-moralistic over public health statements) prevailed in every location; only in Istanbul and Paris did the proportion of responses endorsing a nonpunitive orientation approach that endorsing the punitive.

In terms of attribute categories, more responses were "nonjudgmental" than "judgmental," "optimistic" than "pessimistic," and congruent with data generally accepted by competent authorities rather than "distorted" (in ratios of approximately 11:9, 16:9, and 16:9 respectively).

Statistically significant differences among these second sets of responses were at least as much a function of socioeconomic class and degree of expertise as of geographic location; age and sex were not generally significant discriminators.[3] Judgmental, pessimistic, and distorted responses were significantly more common among lower-class and uninformed, uninvolved subjects, and significantly less common among upper-class subjects and experts. The proportion of responses considered judgmental was also endorsed in amounts significantly higher than the mean in Athens and Bombay (and to a lesser extent in Dublin), whereas respondents in Istanbul and Paris were significantly *less* likely to endorse such responses. Similarly, the proportion of responses involving pessimistic and distorted attributes was endorsed in amounts significantly higher than the mean by respondents in Athens and Dublin for the former, and Athens and Bombay for the latter, while a proportion of responses in amounts significantly below the mean was found among respondents in Paris and Istanbul for the former, and Paris

---

[3]That this finding is not an artifact of the research method is supported by the responses to the first major interview topic—the most serious crimes—in which significant differences were primarily a function of geographic location, rather than of socioeconomic class or degree of expertise (see Weiss and Perry [12]).

Table 1
Total Numbers of Respondents Endorsing Various Strategies for Dealing with Crime and Criminals (N=258)

Category	Percentage
Problem-solving approach—a considered suggestion indicating or implying some way of dealing with crime or criminals in an organized, step-by-step manner	65.5
Emphasis on traditional (retrograde, static) values—need for remaining with or returning to older beliefs and processes, as defined in twentieth-century Western civilization (including traditional religious values)	34.9
Emphasis on rehabilitation, re-education, or treatment—enabling the offender through some process to return to a useful and/or non-criminal role in society (includes changes in probation and parole procedures)	27.5
Emphasis on social prevention—general social program to prevent or reduce crime, directly or indirectly (includes changes in police, judicial, and/or prison systems)	25.6
Moralistic emphasis—emotional, intolerant reaction to deviance of any kind	25.2
Emphasis on punishment	18.6
a. Concern for abstract justice—prescribed punishments for categorized crimes—"an eye for an eye"	11.2
b. Punishment for punishment's sake	7.4
Emphasis on need for more information, data, or research	9.7
Emphasis on "social" portection—a desire to protect the community from crime or its effects through specific defense measures (e.g., more police patrols)	5.8
Misapplication or differential application of selected information—utilizing various bits of information inappropriately or illogically to make a point	3.9
Concern only for humaneness, with no other elements present (includes opposition to capital punishment without justification and without indication of any other content category)	3.5
Emphasis on individual prevention—suggestions for specific preventive measures for particular individuals prior to the commission of a crime (e.g., foster homes for high-risk adolescents)	2.7
Emphasis on individual deterrence—indication that punishment corrects or cures	1.6
Emphasis on "social" deterrence—suggestion that offender should be dealt with in such a way as to discourage others from committing crimes (e.g., "make an example of the criminal")	1.2
Idiosyncratic or not otherwise classified content (miscellaneous content categories endorsed by less than one percent of respondents per category)	1.6

and St. Louis for the latter. A pattern thus begins to form, with the statements of lower-class and uninformed persons, as well as those in Athens, Bombay, and Dublin, tending to be significantly more judgmental, pessimistic, and distorted than the average, and the statements of upper-class persons and experts, and those in Paris and Istanbul, tending to be significantly less so.

Statistically significant differences among response *content* categories demonstrated a division of the various demographic subgroups toward the two orientation models noted earlier. The proportion of responses emphasizing a problem-solving approach was significantly higher among expert and upper-class respondents and significantly lower for uninformed and lower-class respondents. That is, although the problem-solving approach was endorsed heavily by all groups, more experts and upper-class subjects and fewer uninformed and lower-class respondents than the average emphasized this variable. The reservoir of traditional-moralistic opinions was clearly to be found among middle-class and especially lower-class and uninformed, uninvolved persons, and those in Athens, Bombay, and (to a lesser extent) Dublin. Conversely, experts, upper-class respondents, and those in Paris and Istanbul endorsed such content categories significantly below the mean. Only the uninformed significantly emphasized an "eye-for-an-eye" concern; only lower-class subjects and older persons significantly emphasized punishment for punishment's sake; and only uninformed, uninvolved persons paid any significant attention to the importance of deterrence.

On the other hand, the proportion of responses emphasizing the need for more information, data, or research was significantly higher than the mean especially among involved persons and upper-class respondents, and somewhat less so among experts and those in Tokyo. Endorsement of general or specific programs of social protection was highest among experts, the young, and respondents in London, while programs of rehabilitation, re-education, and treatment were most commonly endorsed by upper-class persons. Endorsement of general social programs of prevention was especially high among young and middle-aged persons, men, and respondents in Paris, Istanbul, and St. Louis, while older persons, women, and those in Bombay, Tokyo, and Athens significantly underendorsed this variable. Finally, idiosyncratic responses (although rare by definition) were found primarily among older persons, women, and respondents in Istanbul.

Thus, a pattern of significant differences among the various demographic subgroups in terms of response content categories also becomes apparent. In general, the traditional-moralistic orientation (static, intolerant, punitive) is most common among lower-class persons; uninformed, uninvolved persons; and those in Athens, Bombay, and Dublin. Those emphasizing more strongly the public health orientation (concern with problem-solving, need for more information, social programs for change, and rehabilitation) are more commonly found among experts, upper-class persons, and those living in Paris or Istanbul—although the group with this latter orientation is somewhat smaller in number and somewhat more diffuse in the nature of their opinions than the former. Nevertheless, there appeared to be a considerable degree of confusion, inconsistency, and overlap among all groups. Except for the strong endorsement of a problem-solving approach by almost two-thirds of the subjects, nowhere was there the same clear concensus that existed among the same subjects in defining homicide, theft, and other forms of violent offenses as the "worst" crimes.

DISCUSSION

At this time in history, crime is viewed by a majority of persons in large urban areas throughout the world as one of the most serious social problems, and people appear to be most concerned about homicide and other crimes of violence, theft, and exploitation and public dishonesty. People also believe that they know what to do about crime: Almost all of our subjects made confident recommendations prescribing some definite course of action, policy, or direction. Almost two-thirds endorsed a problem-solving approach; dealing with crime in an organized step-by-step manner is the most common perceived strategy for control.

But opinions as to what those organized steps should be are polarized, confused, and contradictory. Somewhat fewer people tend to give responses that are judgmental, pessimistic, or distorted than otherwise, but somewhat more people tend to endorse a traditional, moralistic, punitive orientation rather than one that emphasizes a public health model (in which crime is regarded as a social illness to be dealt with through programs of primary, secondary, and tertiary prevention).

Such attitudes appear to be related mostly to socioeconomic class, degree of expertise and experience, and geographic location; age and sex are not generally significant discriminators here. Lower-class (and to a lesser extent middle-class) persons, the uninformed and uninvolved, and those in certain cities (Athens, Bombay, and Dublin in this study) are significantly more likely to endorse judgmental, pessimistic, traditional, and punitive strategies. Upper-class persons, experts, and those in other cities (especially Paris and Istanbul in this study) are significantly more likely to endorse problem-solving, preventive, and rehabilitative strategies, albeit somewhat more diffusely.

Persons in the middle socioeconomic class, middle age group, and the other cities in this study (London, St. Louis, and Tokyo) tend as well to have opinions in the middle range—similar to those of the subject group as a whole, more traditional-moralistic than otherwise. Persons categorized as "special interest" or "involved" are unique in some aspects, however. Defined as those who have had some personal or occupational involvement with crime or criminals (or whose spouse, parent, child, or sibling is so involved) but who are clearly *not* experts, this group consisted mostly of lower-ranking policemen and other workers in the law-enforcement, forensic, and penal systems, or their first-degree relatives (55 percent), a number of respondents who had actually committed crimes or their first-degree relatives (38 percent), and some victims—or close relatives of victims—of crime (7 percent). This diverse group was characterized by a generally neutral orientation, but strongly endorsed the need for more information, data, or research, and significantly underendorsed the need for general or specific programs of social protection. In other words, the persons closest to the action, whether as policemen, criminals, or victims, seem to want most more facts, more careful analysis, and more knowledge before proceeding to action programs, especially those deemed "protective."

Despite the apparent perceptions of some politicians, most people (including those directly involved with crime and criminals) endorse a problem-solving approach. Only uninformed, uninvolved persons put much genuine faith in an "eye-for-an-eye" ethic or the usefulness of deterrence. Punitive orientations are more popular than nonpunitive, but not just punishment for punishment's sake. The rationale for the punitive orientation, other than traditional values, seems vague in most people's minds. On the other hand, many of those who support a public health model are hard put to offer concrete, cohesive strategies, and a substantial minority provide confused and internally contradictory suggestions. Despite the documented success of certain crime-prevention programs (decriminalization of some "victimless" offenses; higher salaries, more selective recruitment, and better training for police; gun control; increased use of proven technical aids such as scan-and-search at airports; home and business security systems; and better lighting in slum areas at night—just a few of those now available), that success is either unknown, ignored, or disliked by most respondents (including some "experts" in our sample). The thoughtful analyses and clearly reasoned proposals of such authors as Menninger (20) and Morris and

Hawkins (21) appear to have had relatively little impact.

Rehabilitation—enabling the offender through some process such as re-education or treatment to return to a useful or at least noncriminal role in society—requires special mention. Despite widespread current criticism, this strategy was endorsed by more than a quarter of respondents, most strongly by the better-educated, upper-socioeconomic-class subjects. Many subjects who supported this approach stated that it had never been given a fair chance: Resources and personnel to this end were woefully inadequate, and attempts in most institutions were doomed to failure by the antitherapeutic, custodial, punitive nature of the environment. Indeed, in one country respondents noted that "rehabilitation center" was a notorious euphemism for a particularly brutal kind of punitive detention camp.

Members of the lower socioeconomic classes, however, endorsed the rehabilitation strategy significantly *less* than the average, and yet it is from this group that a very substantial majority of convicted felons come (22, 23). A self-fulfilling prophecy would seem to operate here. Guze (23), having demonstrated that "sociopathy, alcoholism, and drug dependence are the psychiatric disorders characteristically associated with serious crime," then argues that treatment for these crime-associated psychiatric conditions is not at present "consistently and predictably effective," and suggests that "unless more effective procedures are developed for rehabilitating convicted criminals . . . imprisonment until middle age, at least for recidivist criminals, should result in a major reduction in recidivism after discharge from prison. This course of action, if adopted, would be justified by the pessimism surrounding current rehabilitation practices and accomplishments."

Such an actuarial approach, superficially appealing, has in fact many defects. First of all, the data presented here indicate that substantial numbers of better-educated people in large cities scattered throughout the world are *not* pessimistic about current (and especially potential) "rehabilitation practices and accomplishments." (Even if they were, such pessimism would no more justify discarding a process that some studies have demonstrated to be effective under certain conditions—see Morris and Hawkins (21)—than the pessimism and doubt about vaccination against smallpox in 1797 would have justified throwing out that procedure.) Second, Guze's own data indicate that there would be a large number of false positives; i.e., as many as 40 percent of young offenders who otherwise would never commit another crime would be kept in prison for as many as 20 years or more. Third, Morris (24) has provided cogent arguments that such a tactic is unjust, inhumane, and probably unconstitutional.[4]

Does rehabilitation carry any real promise then? The analogy to psychiatric treatment of low-income groups may be instructive. Since the investigations of Hollingshead and Redlich (19) published in 1958, numerous other studies have also supported the contentions that (a) "the evidence is unambiguous and powerful that the lowest social classes have the highest rates of severe psychiatric disorder in our society" (25), and (b) members of the lower socioeconomic classes are more likely to hold negative attitudes toward treatment, especially that based on dynamically oriented psychotherapy (19). Yet Lorion (26) has reported "findings [that] indicated that *some* members of these low-income groups can respond quite positively to psychotherapy" (italics ours). Moreover, Lorion cites other studies presenting evidence "that as treatment procedures are made more responsive to their life styles and needs, [lower-class patients] increasingly begin to use and benefit from mental health

---

[4]Guze's (23) rigorous and extensive investigation may contain one other inferential misconstruction. He studied 223 consecutive convicted male criminals and 66 similar females in Missouri. Using systematic criteria for diagnosis, with well-designed interview techniques for both the subjects and their first-degree relatives, as well as long-term follow-up investigation, he demonstrated that more than half of his subjects were clearly sociopathic and at least a quarter were clearly suffering from alcoholism, with substantial overlap. But Guze repeatedly cites drug dependence as the third of "the big three," although his own data make this conclusion less tenable. Only 10 men and 16 women were definitely drug-dependent (and in the case of the women, the diagnostic criteria appear to have been somewhat different). In addition, the study of female felons began about 10 years after the study of males, making the possibility of differential sociolegal patterns of arrest and conviction solely for drug-related offenses more likely. (No male index crime was listed as a drug violation, but 10 of the female index crimes were.) *All* of the drug-dependent male felons were sociopaths, as were 13 of the 16 women so described. That is, only a minority of the sociopaths was drug-dependent, but no male offender and only three female offenders were drug-dependent without also meeting the diagnostic criteria for sociopathy. Thus, Guze's data certainly support sociopathy and alcoholism, both independently and synergistically, as the major psychiatric conditions associated with most non-white-collar crime, but the evidence from that study itself supports drug dependence only as an occasional complicating factor among sociopathic felons.

facilities." Thus lower-class offenders, more likely to have the highest rates of conviction for crime and at the same time to hold the most negative attitudes toward rehabilitation and treatment procedures, do in *some* cases respond quite positively to such procedures, and may well do so more commonly and more durably if rehabilitation is made "more responsive to their life styles and needs."

Psychiatrists and other health professionals (members of the upper-socioeconomic and expert classes by our definitions) are thus most likely to endorse nonpunitive preventive, rehabilitative, and therapeutic strategies. They must expect antagonism, not only from the offenders themselves, but from the larger body of lower- and middle-class, uninformed and uninvolved persons who endorse more traditional, punitive approaches. It has been shown that a majority of people, and especially upper-class and expert respondents, wants an organized, problem-solving, step-by-step strategy. To help provide it, perhaps more psychiatrists must join the group most emphasizing the need for more information, data, and research—those who are involved.

SUMMARY

Viewing criminal behaviors as sociopsychiatric phenomena clearly influenced by cultural norms and values that define which behaviors are considered deviant, we utilized a small-sample model to determine relevant qualitative attributes of public opinion among subjects in eight large cities scattered throughout the world. Our results indicate that people in urban areas are somewhat more likely to endorse a traditional, moralistic, punitive orientation to social control of crime than otherwise, although a majority want an organized, problem-solving approach. Significant differences among respondents are related especially to social-class, educational, and experience variables; upper-class persons and experts tend to endorse strongly preventive and rehabilitative strategies. Implications bearing upon psychiatric and criminological treatment and disposition processes are discussed.

REFERENCES

1. Scheff, T.J. The societal reaction to deviance: Ascriptive elements in the psychiatric screening of mental patients in a mid-western state. *Soc. Problems*, 11: 401–413, 1964.

2. Skolnick, J.H. *Justice without Trial: Law Enforcement in Democratic Society.* New York: Wiley, 1966.
3. Langley, M.H. The juvenile court: The making of a delinquent. *Law Society Rev.,* 7: 273–298, 1972.
4. McCartney, J.L. A review of recent research in delinquency and deviance. *J. Operat. Psychiat.,* 5: 52–68, 1974.
5. Törnudd, P. Search for causes—the cul-de-sac of criminology. *Sosiologia* (Helsinki), 1: 1–11 (Report No. 3), 1969.
6. Mäkelä, K. Public sense of justice and judicial practice. *Acta Sociologica* (Copenhagen), 10: 1–27, 1966.
7. Hogarth, J. *Sentencing as a Human Process.* Toronto: University of Toronto Press, 1971.
8. Bohmer, C. Judicial attitudes toward rape victims. *Judicature,* 57: 303–307, 1974.
9. Watson, N.A., and Sterling, J.W. *Police and Their Opinions.* Washington, D.C.: International Association of Chiefs of Police, 1969.
10. Murdock, G.P. *Social Structure.* New York: Macmillan, 1949.
11. Weiss, J.M.A., and Perry, M.E. Transcultural attitudes toward homicide and suicide. *Suicide,* 5: 223–227, 1975.
12. Weiss, J.M.A., and Perry, M.E. Transcultural attitudes toward antisocial behavior: The "worst" crimes. *Soc. Sci. Med.,* 10: 541–545, 1976.
13. Thompson, G.C. The evaluation of public opinion. In *Reader in Public Opinion and Communication,* ed. B. Berelson and M. Janowitz. Glencoe, Ill.: Free Press, 1955.
14. Stephenson, W. Application of Q to the assessment of public opinion. Columbia, Mo.: University of Missouri, 1968 (mimeographed).
15. Stephenson, W.: Application of Q-method to the measurement of public opinion. *Psychol. Rec.,* 14: 265–273, 1964.
16. Stephenson, W.: Application of the Thompson schema to the current controversy over Cuba. *Psychol. Rec.,* 14: 275–290, 1964.
17. Stephenson, W. *The Play Theory of Mass Communication.* Chicago: University of Chicago Press, 1967.
18. Stephenson, W. *The Study of Behavior.* Chicago: University of Chicago Press, 1953.
19. Hollingshead, A.B., and Redlich, F.C. *Social Class and Mental Illness.* New York, Wiley, 1958.
20. Menninger, K.A. *The Crime of Punishment.* New York: Viking Press, 1968.
21. Morris, N., and Hawkins, G. *The Honest Politician's Guide to Crime Control.* Chicago: University of Chicago Press, 1970.
22. Wolfgang, M.E. *Patterns in Criminal Homicide.* Philadelphia: University of Pennsylvania Press, 1958.
23. Guze, S.B. *Criminality and Psychiatric Disorders.* New York: Oxford University Press, 1976.

24. Morris, N. The future of imprisonment: Toward a punitive philosophy. *Michigan Law Rev.*, 72: 1161–1180, 1974.
25. Fried, M. Social differences in mental health. In: *Poverty and Health: A Sociological Analysis*, ed. J. Kosa, A. Antonovsky, and I.K. Zola. Cambridge, Mass.: Harvard University Press, 1969.
26. Lorion, R.P. Mental health treatment of the low-income groups. *Contemp. Issues Mental Health*, 1: 1–53, 1975.

Part II
CURRENT RESEARCH IN CULTURAL PSYCHIATRY IN THE UNITED STATES

Introduction

RONALD M. WINTROB

The terms transcultural psychiatry and cross-cultural psychiatry have come into use in the past 20 years to identify a field of investigation of the relation between culture and mental illness. The field of inquiry focused initially and primarily on the differences in manifest behavior—in symptomatology—between individuals in Western countries defined as mentally ill and those in the developing countries. It was a comparative-psychopathology focus, the point of reference being Western psychiatric description and classification. From a starting point of describing differences in symptomatology, research has increasingly been directed toward those cultural factors that could be contributory or even causative of mental illness, as well as those that might be related to the alleviation or prevention of mental illness.

More recently there has been an emergence of what might be called the intracultural study of deviant and disturbed behavior.

69

Here the objective is not to compare the appearance of mental illness in two countries or cultures, but to determine the conceptual and descriptive categories of disturbed behavior within one culture, as defined by the people themselves. This perspective involves clarification of culturally shared beliefs and values relevant to the maintenance of health and the causes of illness. Another term used to define this sphere of investigation is ethnopsychiatry; or more broadly, ethnomedicine. Another trend in cultural research in recent years has been the turning of attention from developing to developed countries, the purpose being to describe the beliefs, attitudes, and behaviors of defined ethnic or cultural groups within countries such as the United States toward mental illness, its treatment and prevention. As a consequence of these developments, the dimensions of the field of cultural psychiatry have become clearer and methods of research have evolved that are more congruent with the research objectives.

The papers in this section clearly reflect the broadening perspective of cultural-psychiatry research currently in progress in the United States. Taken as a group, the papers are concerned with psychosocial stresses affecting American Indians and Eskimos, Puerto Ricans and blacks, as well as a group of recently arrived Vietnamese. They address the issues of intracultural definition of disturbed behavior and intercultural differences in such behavior, as well as attitudes toward treatment and experiences with treatment both by folk healers within the community and by psychiatric serices from outside.

The section begins with a paper by Shore reviewing his experiences in mental health consultation with Indian tribes of the Northwest during the past 10 years. Shore is particularly concerned with the relevance and utilization of research data consonant with community involvement in and sanction of studies of the mental health problems of Indian communities. He points out that intertribal differences in mental health problems require divergent strategies for intervention, and illustrates this with reference to problems of school dropouts, alcohol abuse, and attempted suicide.

Another and complementary assessment of violent behavior is reported by Kraus and Buffler. Their paper examines the statistics for violent death in Alaska during the past 25 years. They demonstrate striking differences in statistics for deaths due to accidents, alcoholism, suicide, and homicide between the Native Alaskan population of Eskimos, Indians, and Aleuts as compared with the non-Native population. Kraus and Buffler's data show that during the past 10 years deaths by accident and alcohol-related deaths have increased among non-Natives, while suicide and homicide have decreased. By contrast, violent death among Alaskan Natives during the same period has steadily increased in all four categories.

Following these two papers concerning American Indians and Eskimos, contributions by Ruiz and Griffith and by Wintrob focus on the Hispanic population of the United States, with particular reference to Puerto Ricans and black Americans. Ruiz and Griffith describe the system of beliefs in spell-casting or hex, and spirit possession or *espiritismo* commonly encountered among Puerto Ricans. They cite two case examples from their clinical experience of Puerto Rican patients in whom beliefs in hex and spirit possession play a central role. They then discuss a number of criteria or guidelines to help psychiatrists evaluate the clinical significance of their patients' beliefs and determine an effective plan of management.

Wintrob's paper reviews the systems of folk beliefs known to many blacks and Hispanics which distinguish between disordered behavior—and physical complaints—believed to be naturally caused, and illnesses believed to be unnaturally induced. Wintrob discusses the significance of these beliefs in spiritism and malign magic or rootwork in determining selection of treatment procedures and attitudes toward effective care.

The section concludes with a paper by Yamamoto and his colleagues at the University of Southern California outlining the stresses and early adaptational problems being experienced by a group of Vietnamese who have migrated to the United States at the end of the Vietnam war, in many cases leaving members of their families behind in Southeast Asia.

Psychiatric Research Issues With American Indians

JAMES H. SHORE

This paper explores issues in transcultural psychiatric research with American Indians with a focus on the relevance and utilization of research outcome. The recent emphasis on Indian community sponsorship of health services and increased activity within the field of Indian mental health has focused attention on mental health evaluation. These issues raise significant questions for all health professionals involved in transcultural psychiatric research.

What community sanctions are appropriate in planning and implementing mental health research?

Who is in control of the research project and the distribution of the findings?

What is the relevance of mental health research to the Indian community?

I began my mental health work with American Indian communities in the 1960's as a consultant for a village on the Pacific Northwest coast. The tribe was part of the Northwest cultural group. From this initial consultation project which involved clinical services and psychiatric epidemiology, I later expanded my involvement with Indian programs to a full-time commitment. I became the director of a regional mental health program for all tribes in the Pacific Northwest under the sponsorship of the Indian Health Service, a branch of the U.S. Public Health Service. At the same time I coordinated the development of a national research program within the eight area mental health programs of the Indian Health Service. This experience in mental health research with American Indian communities involved projects in suicidology, alcohol-treatment effectiveness, Indian boarding schools, and child-care programs. The difficult questions cited above were debated from the beginning of each research proposal. In this paper, I shall report on the findings from several projects in transcultural psychiatric research and review the outcomes in the context of the issues concerning community sanction and relevance of data utilization by the local Indian community.

GUIDELINES FOR INDIAN RESEARCH

In developing mental health research for the Indian Health Service, the staff established a set of informal guidelines which attempted to deal with the increasing criticisms being heard from Indian communities as they voiced concern about previous experiences with social scientists. These guidelines grew out of experience in working with many American Indian tribes from all regions of the country.

1. Planning for mental health projects should begin with collaboration between the social scientist and the Indian community.

2. The focus for a particular research project should be compatible with local priorities of the tribal council or community health committee.

3. In the research design and selection of a particular methodology, consideration should be given to the relevance of the outcome for use by the Indian group.

4. The project should be implemented in a partnership with the local community with an attempt to employ Indian staff whenever possible.

5. An agreement should involve sharing the research findings with the local community in a manner that would maximize relevance for program planning and development.

6. If human subjects are involved, patient rights must be protected. The newly created American Indian and Alaskan Native Research and Development Center (1) has recently stated their concern for these issues by issuing a patient bill of rights.

RESEARCH IN SUICIDOLOGY

With regard to suicides among American Indians, our research demonstrated that the stereotype of the suicidal Indian is a misconception overlooking the tribal-specific nature of the suicide pattern (2). Suicide rates vary significantly among different tribes. The annual rate ranges from 8 to over 100 per 100,000, documenting the importance of the tribal-specific nature of self-destructive behavior which should not be represented as "an American Indian problem." These data were used in consultation with tribal health committees to clarify the non-Indian misconception of "the suicidal Indian" which had been incorporated as an Indian belief. This misconception had several consequences: first, it involved misunderstandings based on an assumption that all American Indians have identical health problems and consequently similar suicide patterns and rates; second, it failed to recognize the importance of tribal differences for health patterns; and third, it presented a danger that public health personnel were not specific with individual high-risk tribes in designing programs for crisis intervention. In a recent consultation with the tribal health committee of a large Southwest tribe, I had the experience of hearing the tribal leader emphasize their "Indian suicide problem." The tribal health council was convinced, because of public news media reports, that suicide was their major mental health problem. As a non-Indian consultant, I was in the unique position of pointing out their suicide was strikingly low as compared with some tribes and perhaps no higher than non-Indian rates. A non-Indian misconception had been incorporated as an Indian belief, a misconception that carried with it a negative self-image for that particular Indian community and the loss of self-esteem by tribal members.

Additional research in suicidology has demonstrated that recent acculturation pressures for tribes of the Northern Great Plains and groups of Alaskan Natives and Indians have been associated with a dramatic rise in suicide rates. Within high-risk communities it has been possible to identify specific high-risk subgroups along extended family lines. These data provide the opportunity to plan for preventive programs in mental health. With this information, however, a new danger exists of labeling a small number of Indian tribes with the suicidal Indian stereotype and then stigmatizing individual tribal members as high risk. As the identification of high-risk tribes and individual subgroups has become possible, the capacity to identify those in need of help has exceeded our potential to respond effectively with program implementation. It is important that these findings, along with limitations in our current mental health delivery systems, be clearly explained to Indian communities.

ALCOHOL PROGRAM RESEARCH

In an independent investigation effort, we evaluated the treatment effectiveness of a regional Indian alcohol program (3) that had been developed to serve major tribes of the Pacific Northwest. Follow-up data were collected by an Indian counselor and a psychiatrist on 83 American Indian alcoholic men. The follow-up status was judged by an interdisciplinary panel according to a six-step rating scale. The improvement rate compared favorably with other treatment programs, especially in view of the selection process for this regional treatment center, which favored difficult patients. The findings documented successful treament outcomes for more than one-third of the clients. The report was used to justify contract medical funds for alcohol rehabilitation. This research outcome demonstrated that a history of arrest among Indian male alcoholics was not a negative predictor of treatment outcome. The information supported an open admission policy and gave encouragement to the staffs who treated patients with chronic, recurrent drinking problems.

The interracial, interdisciplinary rating panel was developed as an evaluation method that would provide a check for erroneous judgment of Indian drinking status. Levy and Kunitz (4) have discussed this problem in detail: "numerous difficulties which have plagued the data-gathering process in studies of American Indian drinking, while they remain with us, may be overcome to a great extent by the use of more uniform methods of investigation, explicit definitions, and whenever possible by a multidisciplinary approach. As long as the methods of one discipline remain unchecked by the use of other methods, erroneous interpretations of the findings will be unnecessarily frequent." However, after reporting this project, our approach gained little acceptance either in the local community or with national consultants who were developing evaluation methods for Indian alcohol programs. In part, we felt that the resistance to an interracial, interdisciplinary rating panel was not related to this specific research method, but was caused by the difficulty in bridging the gap between mental health and alcohol programs. More specifically, this difficulty is created by a separation between paraprofessional alcohol counselors and professional mental health workers. The interaction of the professional staff, who operate from a scientific model, with the paraprofessional worker, whose model of treatment has followed craft lines, has created unique problems and tensions (5).

RESEARCH IN INDIAN BOARDING SCHOOLS

A research project in an Indian boarding school focused on the high-risk student group for school dropout (6). This student body and school staff had experienced increased stress over a four-year period that became manifest as an eightfold increase in the dropout rate between 1967 and 1971. During this time the dropout rate rose from three to 26 percent of the entire student body. A systematic research project was conducted to evaluate student records from both a dropout and nondropout group. Multiple sociocultural items were identified in the student's background that were significantly related to subsequent dropping out of school. At the same time, several distinct new mental health programs were initiated with the goal of decreasing the dropout rate. The research and subsequent program development were done in collaboration with the student body, school staff, and Indian school board. In the first year following the development of the new programs, the school dropout rate was lowered from 26 to 19 percent of the student body. In subsequent years, however, the school board and administration did not utilize the information to systematically identify high-risk students.

The disappointing experience of this incomplete boarding school consultation has often been reported by other mental health consultants in many areas of the country. Both Bergman and Goldstein (7) and Hammerschlag et al. (8) have separately reported their experiences in consultation with the Southwestern American Indian boarding schools. Repeated frustrations of mental health professionals who are working within boarding school programs reflect a conflict between the psychiatric consultant who is working to develop specific programs for high-risk students and the Bureau of Indian Affairs educational staff, who do not want to compromise educational priorities by turning boarding schools into "treatment settings." With the recent growth of the Indian advisory school boards, attention has focused on issues of Indian control and cultural identity. While these various goals are not conflicting, the consulting experience of many psychiatrists in working within the boarding school system has been similar. The multiple resistances which block an effective utilization of evaluation outcome in this and other boarding school settings are crucial issues to consider as future research projects are proposed.

RESEARCH OF INDIAN CHILD-CARE NEEDS

In a program-development consultation with a tribe of Northwest Plateau Indians, we developed a community-based children's home and child welfare program (9). The program was effective because of its compatibility with Indian culture which accepted extended family and community responsibility for child care. In the first 18 months of operation, the tribal child-care program reduced the annual placements of Indian children in off-reservation foster care from 35 to one. This preliminary evaluation of a child-care program supported a rationale of primary prevention in community mental health. The program prevented off-reservation placement of Indian children. These results have been used in consultation with numerous Indian leaders who are concerned with similar issues of child welfare and foster-home placement. However, this is a simple standard of evaluation that does not compare long-term criteria which might assess the psychological adjustment of Indian children following placement in multiple settings.

DISCUSSION

An unavoidable conclusion from these examples of transcultural psychiatric research is the implied limitation on the freedom of the social scientist in research inquiry. This issue cannot be passed over lightly. Can research priorities be subjected to Indian community and political control without seriously compromising the nature of scientific inquiry? My own resolution of this dilemma leads to a strong conviction that the social scientist must consider the issues of community involvement, participation, and shared control. Just as individual patient rights are protected by human subject regulations, community rights among American Indians must be respected. An involved mental health professional can openly debate a disagreement with Indian representatives and sometimes change their approach. However, one must proceed with caution since Indian group wisdom, stated for protection of their vested interest, is usually as accurate as the so-called scientific world view. An obvious approach to this dilemma lies in the involvement of more American Indian researchers, who, nevertheless, will face problems similar to those of the non-Indian social scientist as the Indian professionals work with their own people.

SUMMARY

In this paper I have identified several significant issues in transcultural psychiatric research with American Indians and focused on the relevance and utilization of research outcome. Complex questions are raised by the current emphasis on Indian community sponsorship and increased research activity in the field of mental health. I have drawn from my experiences in psychiatric research with American Indians and reported on specific projects in suicidology, alcohol-treatment effectiveness, Indian boarding schools, and child-care programs. In *Custer Died for Your Sins*, Vine Delorio (10) presented a clear warning to all health professionals when he singled out anthropologists as a paradigm for criticism: "Anthropologists come out to the Indian reservations to make observations. During the winter these observations will become books by which future anthropologists will be trained so that they can come out to reservations years from now and verify the observations they have studied" (p. 79). The message is clear. The relevance of future transcultural psychiatric research with American Indians will be judged by that standard.

REFERENCES

1. Fowler, H., et al. American Indian Bill of Rights. Declaration by the White Cloud Center, American Indian and Alaskan Native Research and Development Center, Portland, Oregon, 1976 (mimeographed).
2. Shore, J.H. American Indian suicide—fact and fantasy. *Psychiatry*, 38: 86–89. 1975.
3. Wilson, L.G., and Shore, J.H. Evaluation of a regional Indian alcohol program. *Amer. J. Psychiat.*, 132: 255–258, 1975.
4. Levy, J.E., and Kunitz, S.J. Indian drinking problems of data collection and interpretation. Presented at the first annual conference of the National Institute of Alcohol Abuse and Alcoholism, Washington, D.C., June 25–26, 1971.
5. Kalb, M., and Propper, M.S. The Future of alcohology: Craft or science? *Amer. J. Psychiat.*, 133: 6, 1976.
6. Shore, J.H. Preventive mental health programs for American Indian youth—success and failure. In: *Mental Health in Children*, ed. D.V. Siva Sankar 1: 61–71. Westbury, N.Y.: PJD Publications, 1975.
7. Bergman, R.L., and Goldstein, G.S. The model dorm: Changing Indian

boarding schools. Presented at the annual meeting of the American Psychiatric Association, Honolulu, Hawaii, May 7–11, 1973.

8. Hammerschlag, C.A., Clayton, P.A., and Berg, D. Indian education: A human systems analysis. *Amer. J. Psychiat.*, 130: 1098, 1973.

9. Shore, J.H., and Nicholls, W.M. Indian children and tribal group homes; new interpretations of the whipper man. *Amer. J. Psychiat.*, 132: 4, 1975.

10. Deloria, V. *Custer Died for Your Sins*. London: Macmillan, 1969.

7

Intercultural Variation in Mortality Due to Violence

ROBERT KRAUS, M.D.
PATRICIA BUFFLER

Violent behavior in the context of rapid social and cultural change has become a matter of increasing concern in America. This paper deals with one aspect of the problem as observed in the American North, the State of Alaska. We present data illustrating changing patterns of mortality in the various peoples and cultures of Alaska during the interval 1950–1974 with specific reference to deaths due to violence in the form of accidents, suicides, homicides, and alcohol.

ALASKA: AN OVERVIEW

The arctic and subarctic regions make up some 20 percent of the earth's land mass and as the last great frontier and reservoir of untapped natural resources are everywhere undergoing intense exploitation and development. Alaska, whch comprises the American component of these regions, is participating in this process of rapid sociocultural and economic growth and change. The largest state, Alaska encloses approxi-

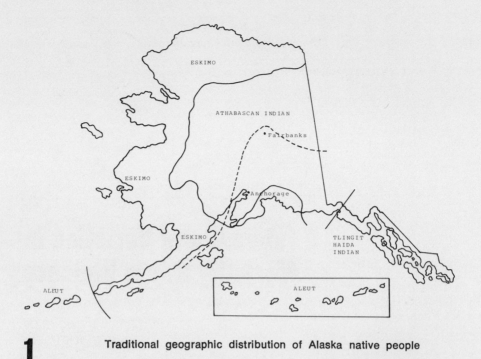

1 Traditional geographic distribution of Alaska native people

mately 580,000 square miles. Within this great area are a series of
different ecological settings ranging from the flat, snow-covered, wind-
swept tundra of the North to the mountains and rain forests of the
Southeast. Interetstingly, the total population of the state in 1974 was
calculated to be 351,075.

Despite its small size, the population of Alaska exhibits striking
social and cultural diversity. Figure 1 illustrates this phenomenon in
part (1). It shows the traditional geographic distribution of the Native
people of Alaska. It is not within the scope of this paper to discuss these
cultures in detail. It should be noted, however, that "Alaskan
Native" is essentially an administrative term which obscures the fact
that Alaska's Eskimos, Indians, and Aleuts are historically, linguistically,
and culturally quite distinct. The non-Native population of Alaska must
be understood in terms of heavy immigration into the state during the
period since 1940. The non-Native population increased sixfold during
that time and began regularly to exceed the Native population in number
only during the period 1940–1950. The dotted diagonal line across the
center of the state depicted in Figure 1 separates Native from non-

Table 1
The Population of Alaska, 1974

Natives ($\underline{N}$=56,861)	
Northern Eskimo	11,842
Western Eskimo	24,255
Athabascan	7,291
Aleut	2,869
Tlingit, Haida, Tsimpshian Indian	10,604
Non-Native ($\underline{N}$=294,214)	
Caucasian	280,215
Black	10,547
Asian-American	3,452
Total	351,075

Native Alaska. North of the line the population is predominantly rural and Native. South of the line it is predominantly urban and non-Native with heavy concentration in the cities of Fairbanks and Anchorage (2). Table 1 summarizes the approximate population figures for the groups mentioned above (3).

CHANGING PATTERNS OF MORTALITY IN ALASKA, 1950–1974

The flow of events outlined above has been accompanied by rather distinctive changes in the patterning of mortality among the various populations in the state. The data presented here represent a synthesis and analysis of a sample of all deaths due to violence in Alaska during the period 1950–1975 as well as relevant data from a variety of sources (4–6).[1]

Figure 2 shows mortality, expressed as percent of total mortality, for the total Alaskan population for selected causes for five year intervals during the period 1950–1974. The general categories for cause of death are: infectious disease; chronic disease, which comprises heart disease, cancer, stroke, and a variety of other chronic diseases usually

[1]Also utilized were various summaries and reports of the Bureau of Vital Statistics, Alaska, and the Alaska Area Native Health Service, as well as certain volumes in the Mortality Series of the National Center for Health Statistics.

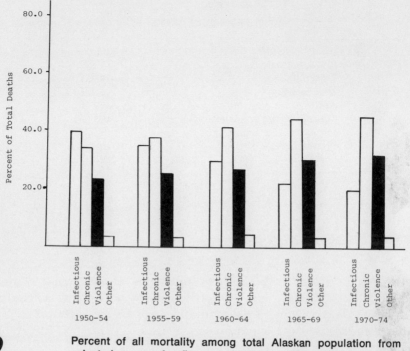

2 Percent of all mortality among total Alaskan population from selected causes for five-year intervals, 1950–1974

classified separately; violent or preventable deaths, which comprise deaths due to accident, suicide, homicide, and alcohol; and deaths due to other causes. It can be seen that deaths due to infectious disease are decreasing and deaths due to chronic disease are increasing, although the percentage of deaths due to chronic disease is significantly lower than that of the total United States pattern. Violent death undergoes a steady increase, until in the most recent interval it comprises in excess of 30 percent of the total picture. It should be noted that the total Alaskan population is heavily weighted toward non-Natives. Only 20 percent of the population is Native.

Figure 3 presents comparable data for the non-Native population of Alaska. This pattern is characterized by an increasing percentage of deaths due to chronic illness, although the percentage remains significantly below the United States (all races) percentage. Apparent again is a high percentage of mortality attributable to violent deaths.

Figure 4 illustrates the mortality pattern for the Native population of Alaska. Striking changes over the last 25 years are evident. Deaths

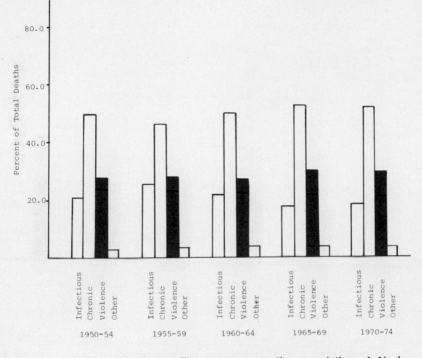

3

Percent of all mortality among non-native population of Alaska from selected causes by five-year intervals, 1950–1974

due to infectious disease have declined precipitously while deaths due to chronic disease have increased, a phenomenon due at least in part to greatly improved medical care. Of particular note is the step-by-step increase in the percentage of violent deaths. During the interval 1950–1954, the percentage of deaths among Natives due to violence was slightly more than half the percentage for non-Natives even though the Natives, by and large, lived in a more dangerous environment. In the more recent intervals the percentage of violent deaths has grown more rapidly for Natives than non-Natives until, in the most recent interval, it constitutes slightly in excess of 40 percent of the total Native mortality.

VIOLENT DEATH IN ALASKA, 1950–1974

Further definition of this emerging problem of death due to violence can be obtained by examining the death rates for each type of violent

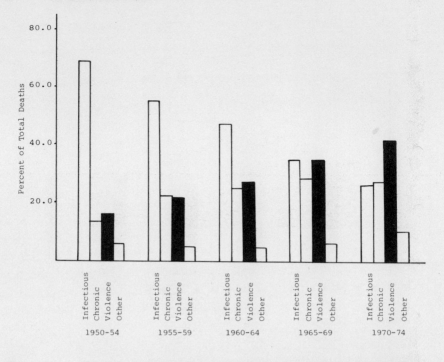

4   Percent of all mortality among Alaskan natives, from selected
causes for five-year intervals, 1950–1974

death—accident, suicide, homicide, and alcohol—for both Natives and
non-Natives for the same time period and comparing the rates to those
of other United States populations.

Figure 5 shows annual accident death rates for Alaskan non-Natives,
Alaskan Natives, total American Indians (including Alaskan Natives),
and the United States (all races). The Alaskan rate seems to be a
manifestation of a phenomenon affecting American Indians generally.
The Alaskan non-Native rate fell during the interval 1950–1964 and has
remained stable although significantly higher than the United States
(all races) rate.

Comparable figures for homicide are summarized in Figure 6.
Current Alaskan Native and American Indian homicide rates are high,
roughly comparable, and reflect an increasing problem of homicide in
the United States generally. It is of interest to note that the Alaskan
non-Native rate has decreased in each time interval and currently is
lower than the United States (all races) rate.

Examination of Figure 7 reveals that the Alaskan Native suicide

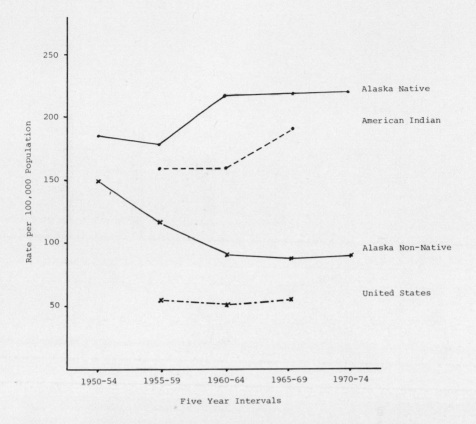

5 Average annual accident death rates for various American populations for five-year intervals, 1950–1974

rate diverged sharply from the American Indian and United States (all races) rates after 1965. As with homicide, the suicide rate for Alaskan non-Natives has decreased steadily since 1950 and is now below the United States (all races) rate.

Deaths due to alcohol present problems of recognition and definition. The alcohol death rates for Alaskan Natives and non-Natives summarized in Figure 8 are based on review and analysis of all alcohol-related deaths recorded by the Bureau of Vital Statistics, Alaska, during 1950–1974. Only those cases coded according to the *International Statistical Classification of Diseases, Injuries, and Causes of Death* (7) as due to alcoholic psychosis, acute alcoholism, chronic alcoholism, alcoholic cirrhosis, or alcohol poisoning as the primary cause of death were

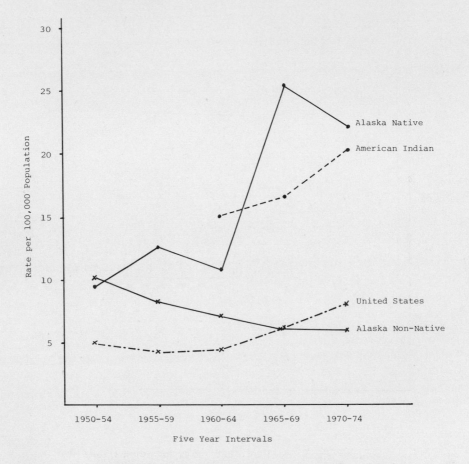

6   Average annual homicide death rates for various American populations for five-year intervals, 1950–1974

utilized. At this time, comparable figures for American Indians and the United States (all races) are being prepared. Deaths due to these causes are increasing in both Natives and non-Natives with the Native increase being more noticeable.

SUMMARY

The data presented above concerning overall patterns of mortality and mortality related to violence are summarized in Table 2 which pre-

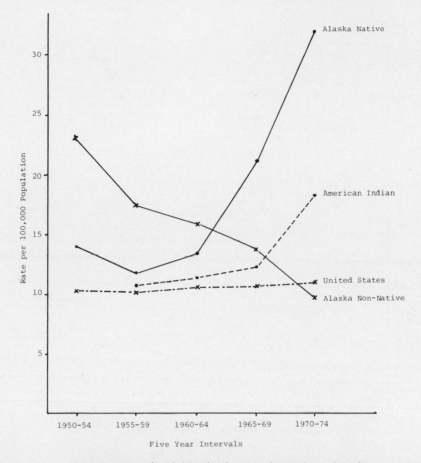

7   Average annual suicide death rates for various American populations for five-year intervals, 1950–1974

sents figures for the year 1970. The familiar United States pattern, mentioned previously, with its large preponderance of deaths due to heart disease, cancer, and stroke is at sharp variance with the Alaskan pattern. Violence, defined as accidents, homicides, sucides, and deaths due to alcohol, is the leading cause of death in Alaska. This is true of both Native and non-Native populations, Among the non-Natives over the last 10 years, the pattern has been maintained by a consistently high rate of death by accident and an increasing rate of deaths due to alcohol. Suicide and homicide are decreasing. Among Natives, the pattern for violent death is related to increases in all four categories.

The people of Alaska therefore constitute a group in which the

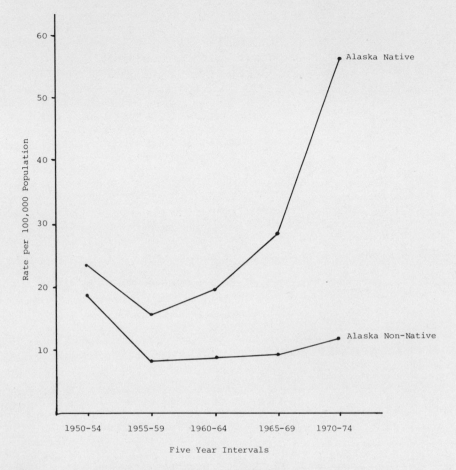

8   Average annual alcohol death rates for Alaska natives and non-natives for five-year intervals, 1950–1974

leading causes of mortality are behaviorally based. This is not a uniform phenomenon; significant intercultural variation in the patterning of mortality exists. The delineation of the psychological, social, and cultural factors underlying this phenomenon is the focus of continuing research.

Presented at the Annual Meeting, American Psychiatric Association Miami, May 1976.

Research supported by National Institutes of Mental Health Research Grants MH 18749 and MH 23233 and the WAMI Program, University of Alaska.

Table 2
Leading Causes of Death Among Alaskan Natives,
All Alaskan Residents and United States, 1970

Rank[a]	Cause	Rate per 100,000 Population		
		Alaskan Natives	Alaska Total	United States
1	Accidents	199.4	116.9	56.4
2	Heart disease	73.0	87.4	362.0
3	Malignant neoplasms	67.1	61.6	162.8
4	Influenza; Pneumonia	49.3	17.9	30.9
5	Alcoholism	41.4	10.9	-
6	Vas. lesions of CNS	35.5	26.2	101.9
7	Disease of early infancy	29.6	25.5	21.3
8	Suicide	29.6	13.2	11.6
9	Homicide	27.6	10.6	8.3

[a]Ranked by order of importance as a cause of death in Alaska Natives.

REFERENCES
1. Oswalt, W. *Alaskan Eskimos*. San Francisco: Chandler, 1967.
2. Federal Field Committee for Development Planning. *Alaska Natives and the Land*. Washington, D.C.: U.S. Government Printing Office, 1968.
3. Buffler, P., and Kraus, R. *Populations and Communities of Alaska*. WAMI Program, University of Alaska, 1976.
4. Frederick, C. *Suicide, Homicide, and Alcoholism Among American Indians*. Washington, D.C.: U.S. Government Printing Office, 1973.
5. Iskrant, A., and Joliet, P. *Accidents and Homicide*. Cambridge, Mass.: Harvard University Press, 1968.
6. Erhardt, C. and Berlin, J. *Mortality and Morbidity in the United States*. Cambridge, Mass.: Harvard University Press, 1974.

8

Hex and Possession: Two Problematic Areas in the Psychiatrist's Approach to Religion

PEDRO RUIZ
EZRA H. GRIFFITH

In the past decade, American psychiatrists have become more sensitive in their treatment of patients who are devout practitioners of and believers in spiritualism. This is partially due to the progressive increase of immigrants coming from countries where spiritualism is encountered. Part of the reason for this increased sensitivity, however, must be American psychiatrists' heightened cognizance of the religious beliefs of these people. Publicity of all sorts has pointed to the presence of these religious practices in our midst; and try as one might, one is unable to disregard the influences these religious beliefs have in shaping the unique and striking manifestations of psychiatric illness among these people. Lubchansky et al. (1), Fisch (2), Ruiz and Langrod (3), and Harwood (4) have argued the logic of psychiatrists' having a solid knowledge of spiritualism if they are to deliver a rational type of mental health care to people who share beliefs in spiritualism and spiritualist practices. There are several problematic areas, however, which hinder the American psychiatrist in being able to grasp the essential features

93

of spiritualism. These areas need to be explored so that the physician is more sensitive to the causes of his frustration when he seems unable to appreciate the intricacies of the beliefs of patients who are spiritualist adherents.

In this paper, while there may be no precise answers given, we shall attempt to elucidate some of these problematic areas in the hope that this additional knowledge will enable the psychiatrist to be better able to assess his patients and arrive at constructive treatment plans. We shall contrast the psychiatrist's and the spiritualist's views of specific phenomena; and by highlighting these differences we hope some clarity will emerge.

The issue of hexing is an old one. Yet it presents one of the most fascinating and complicated problems in the whole history of spiritualism. Simon the Sorcerer (Acts 8) utilized his arts to bewitch the people of Samaria and he became famous for his powers. This is an ancient example of the power of the hex. In psychiatric terms, we can say that the patient is hexed when he believes that his complaint—either somatic or psychic—is caused by the intervention of some being, either human or supernatural. It serves no purpose to consider such patients psychotic because they believe themselves to be hexed. Rather, it is necessary to explore the details of the hex beliefs and attempt to combat them on a level consistent with the patient's understanding. Success is in no way assured at this point in the history of psychiatry.

Hexing is believed to be powerful enough to cause death, and there are cases in the literature which confirm this. Walter Cannon (5) very early opened this area of interesting and exciting research. He observed that among the natives of Australia and New Zealand bone-pointing caused death. The case of Rob is a classic of this genre. Rob has a bone pointed at him by a witch doctor, followed by Rob becoming extremely afraid, distressed, ill, weak. Rob is convinced he will die. When Nebo, the witch doctor, is threatened by a missionary, Nebo decides to save Rob's life. He does it by merely leaning over Rob's bed and telling him that it was all a mistake. Rob quickly recovers.

Cannon believed that for hexing to work to this degree, the person must be primitive and superstitious, with an extremely fertile imagination. He argues that when the subject is so afraid, the sympathico-adrenal system is called into action. This causes a persistent constriction of the small arterioles throughout the body, eventually leading to a reduction in blood pressure, due primarily to a loss of blood volume. The subject then shows all the classic signs of hypovolemic shock with a weak, thready pulse, tachycardia, sweating, coolness, and clamminess of the extremities. The victim will die in cardiac systole; and post-mortem examination would be expected to reveal a heart with practically empty chambers. Consequently Cannon contended that hexing produces a kind of "malignant anxiety" serious enough by involvement of the sympathetic and adrenal systems to produce hypovolemic shock which relentlessly leads to death.

Curt Richter (67) was struck by Cannon's observation, particularly since his own work with rats seemed to contradict Cannon's conclusions. Richter found that the trimming of wild rats' whiskers seemed disturbing enough to cause their deaths. Richter trimmed the whiskers of 12 domesticated rats and then placed them in water at 95°F. Three rats died within two minutes. The remaining nine swam 40 to 60 hours. Most control rats in the 95°F temperature swam 60 to 80 hours. He repeated the experiment with 34 clipped wild rats. All 34 died in less than 15 minutes.

Following Cannon's conclusions, Richter expected the rats to show signs of sympathetic stimulation such as tachycardia, and to die in cardiac systole. Electrocardiographic records, however, indicated that the rats died with a bradycardia. There was also evidence of bradypnea and lowering of body temperature preceding death. At autopsy the rats' hearts were large and distended with blood, indicating death occurred in cardiac diastole. While the initial response of the rats demonstrated tachycardia, prolongation of the stressful situation resulted in definite bradycardia. So instead of the "malignant anxiety" postulated by Cannon, Richter suggested that the stressful situation produced a condition of hopelessness in the rats which seemed to lead to a hyperactivity of the parasympathetic system.

Mathis (7) described the case of a 53-year-old man who had a disagreement with his mother. During the argument, the mother predicted that something would happen to him. Two days later the patient, who had no previous history of respiratory disease, showed signs of bronchial asthma. During the next few months, the patient's relations with his mother worsened and so did his asthma. One day, following a telephone call with his mother in which she had reminded him of her fateful prediction, the patient died. Mathis theorized that the psychophysiological reaction may indeed be a common vehicle for expressing the feeling that one has been hexed.

Cappannari et al. (8) have described a case of hexing and regional enteritis. Here again there is the suggestion that the hex produced psychosocial stress which in turn led to the development or, at least, the worsening of the enteritis.

These four examples describe cases in which the hex is thought to directly produce a somatic or psychosomatic ailment. The somatic issue is a complicated one and we suspect that physicians faced with this type of case would tend to treat it in terms of the observable phenomena. That is, the patient showing the signs of hypovolemic shock would certainly be given fluid replacement, even if it were absolutely clear that the patient attributed the condition to the results of a hex. Similarly, one would expect the hexed patient who presents with marked bronchial constriction to be treated with bronchodilators even in the presence of a history of hexing. But there are two unresolved issues that emerge from this discussion. One relates to the dispute between Cannon and Richter about which system hexing seems to bring into play—the sympathetic or parasympathetic. Unfortunately, Richter can hardly claim that his rats were hexed, and we are still unsure of the degree to which animal experimentation is applicable to humans.

The second issue concerns our willingness to experiment with de-hexing in the face of somatic and psychosomatic complaints when the patient's belief in the etiology of hexing is evident. Such experimentation would indeed be difficult to carry out, particularly in view of the present medicolegal climate in the United States. But one can hardly help wondering what the results of dehexing would be in these cases.

In the psychiatric area, these issues are also coming to the forefront. We have recently encountered two patients in whom belief in hexing clearly contributed to their mental illness. The first was the case of a young Puerto Rican woman who was hospitalized because of bizarre, antisocial behavior. This patient had had an argument with a neighbor who was a practicing spiritualist. The patient, as well as her family, felt sure that the neighbor had put a hex on the patient as a consequence of their verbal conflict. Following the hex episode, the patient gradually began to care less about herself and her children. She started to hear voices which were manipulating her behavior. The voices, as described by the patient, represented spirits and came to the patient principally through a doll, which had itself been given to her by another spiritualist. Accordingly, the patient was convinced that the spiritualist neighbor had converted the doll into a malign symbol, and this was part of the neighbor's plan to drive the patient mad. The patient's relatives, themselves practitioners of and believers in spiritualism, reinforced the patient's concept of her illness. Three psychiatrists had diagnosed this patient as schizophrenic. She was treated with phenothiazines, and at the same time a spiritualist combatted the hex through the performance of a spiritualist ceremony. The patient recovered completely and is now fully functional.

The second case was that of a Puerto Rican woman with a previous history of psychiatric illness, hospitalized because of marked depression and overt suicidal ideation. The patient's husband was an alcoholic who died from gastro-intestinal hemorrhage. Both he and the patient's mother-in-law were avid spiritualists. On the advice of his mother, the husband had once performed a ceremony in which he placed small India ink marks on his wife's face, fingers, buttocks, knees, and breasts. The husband explained that the purpose of the ceremony was to make the wife ugly so that no man would ever look at her again. In addition, the marks represented a symbol of her being indissolubly linked to the husband. In reality, the marks were tiny and hardly noticeable. They were also solitary and not multiple in each specific region.

Following the husband's death, the patient's depression progressively deepened. She felt that the husband still controlled her by virtue of the marks on her skin. She could not envisage a relationship with any other male because of the husband's constant presence. In addition, she was totally convinced that the marks had disfigured her to the point where no man would ever look at her. Consequently, it was useless to live anymore. The patient is still in psychiatric treatment and serious thought is being given to the use of a spiritualist.

DISCUSSION

In the two cases cited, the etiological contribution of the ritualized hex is of obvious importance. Even if the psychiatrist himself doesn't believe in hexing, he must be impressed by the importance that the patient attaches to the phenomenon of hexing. We are no different from other physicians: to treat a diagnosed schizophrenic or depressed patient solely by a dehexing ritual would shock our Westernized psychiatric sensibilities. So we opt for a multiple-level approach to this type of patient. That is, we attempt to counteract the hex through a dehexing process, and we treat the schizophrenic symptomatology with the appropriate tranquilizing drugs.

The situation becomes even more complicated when the symptomatology is less clear and the evidence for a ritualized hex less precise. Mathewson describes Haitian patients who may be merely experiencing the "constraints and angers of illegal immigration status" (9). Because things are going badly for these patients, because they are experiencing overwhelming difficulties in daily living, they attempt to explain it by magical or supernatural means. They rationalize their difficulties by claiming that someone or something is maligning them, or that spirits are punishing them. The question is: How are we to help these patients?

Psychiatric treatment that ignores or derides the spiritualist beliefs of these patients is, in our experience, useless. Yet, these patients don't want to be referred to a spiritualist. They want psychiatric help, not a dehexing experience. There has to be traditional psychotherapy, but with a cultural bias, one that reassures the patient that he can overcome the difficulties presently confronting him. The therapist reduces the chance of helping such patients if he tries to convince them that there are no magical or supernatural influences controlling the patient's life. It is more useful for the therapist to reduce the effects of the patient's generalized belief in hexing through a systematic reinforcement of the patient's ego strengths.

It seems then that hexing is a powerful-enough phenomenon to exert its influences on human beings through somatic, psychic, and psychosomatic mechanisms. It remains unclear why the hex may manifest itself in one patient as bronchial asthma and in another patient as severe depression. There is also some suggestion that one must inherently possess some vulnerability for the hex to be effective. This vulnerability may be characterized by some as genetic, by others as an entity acquired through cultural experience.

The phenomenon of spirit possession is the second problematic area we wish to examine. In the psychiatrist's approach to spiritualism he must understand possession well enough to distinguish between the patient who is possessed and the one who, while having a serious mental illness, claims to be possessed. It is also necessary to understand some of the psychological aspects of spirit possession. Here we speak of spirit possession as existing when there is a relationship between a human being and a spirit such that the spirit has invaded the person and the behavior of the human is said to be that of the spirit.

Haitians (10) speak of the possession as occurring when a *loa* has "mounted" the person; the person is considered the horse that the *loa* rides. Similarly, in *santeria* (11) the saint is said to climb on his horse. The *Shango* worshippers in Trinidad (12) utilize the same concept of the possessed being ridden by a spirit. This notion is important because it communicates clearly the idea that the person is being controlled by some exterior force and, in fact, is no longer responsible for his actions even though certain types of behavior are socially unacceptable.

We have been struck by the amazing similarity of spiritualist possession and the possession rituals observable in many black American Christian churches. In these churches, the devout insist that the Holy Spirit descends and takes over the person, causing the affected individual to sing, dance, and speak in tongues. Indeed, there is some common point in the phenomena of Christian and other forms of spirit possession. We see some evidence of this in the description by Southern (13) of the

Ring Shout performed in the nineteenth century in the United States—women would form a ring, gradually become frenzied, and perform intricate movements while in the throes of religious ecstasy.

The first patient cited earlier, who believed herself to be under the influence of a hex, would repeatedly go into a trance while in hospital, her eyes would roll upward, her arms would move around her body as though she were warding off some invisible opponent, and she would mumble prayers, partly in Spanish, partly in an incomprehensible patois. She would jerk back and forth and the vibrations would increase in intensity, somewhat resembling the convulsions of a seizure state. After a few minutes, she would gradually stop shaking and finally bow in a ritualistic manner indicating that the possession episode had passed. There was no doubt in the minds of her relatives that the patient was undergoing episodic spirit possession. Possession in this case lasted only a few minutes. That seems to be a preferable length of time because it is generally acknowledged that lengthy possession seems to weaken the horse and may indeed lead him finally into madness. While there are reports of people being possessed for several hours at a time, these are invariably initiated priests who seem to tolerate lengthy possession without untoward effects. Similarly, Christian ritual possession occurring during services in church rarely lasts more than a few minutes. The episode may, however, occur several times during the same ceremony. Reports of possession not linked to ceremonial occasions are relatively rare, but such occurrences are related to other unusual situations such as thunderstorms, lightning, or car accidents—all stimuli that may be construed as interventions of the spirits. In the case cited, the patient clearly does not satisfy the requirement of being possessed in habitual circumstances. The place of her possession is inappropriate.

Generally, possessed people are adults ranging in age from 20 to 50, but younger adults are particularly affected. Some spiritualist groups view possession of a child as an indication that the child has been specially chosen by the spirits and will eventually enter the ranks of the priests. Others view child possession as a sign of weakness and believe that such a child is susceptible to mental illness. In the church, a child's being possessed is generally viewed with concern, and there is some question of the authenticity of this type of possession.

There is generally some limitation on nonchurch members witnessing possession rituals, although there is no exclusion of nonbelievers from othere aspects of spiritualist ceremonies. Indeed, the rare examples of spirit possession in public are considered manifestations of punishment by the invading spirit. Once more, the case cited does not satisfy the requirements of secrecy. We have observed that among the people participating in spiritualist practices, the vast majority are women. While there may be a significant number of men present in the black churches, we have also noted that at least two-thirds of those who become possessed are females. Certainly this phenomenon may be partly cultural. It may be culturally more acceptable for women to become disinhibited and possessed. However, when men become possessed, they often take on the roles of women saints. Women also make the sexual transition while posssesed. Possession occurs most easily and swiftly when there is music and most particularly drumming. The rhythm seems to be a powerful stimulant. In the black church, while most possession occurs when there is music, we have also seen it occur during sessions of long, intense praying. The ambience appears enhanced in the presence of incense, candles, a darkened atmosphere, statues, and a cohesive congregation. Our patient's behavior seemed all the more inappropriate in the absence of these stimuli.

We observed that the drummers and musicians who provide the music for the ceremonial occasions rarely undergo possession themselves. Similarly, in the church, the choir director is evidently proud that the music and direction he provides are valuable enough to stimulate the descent of the Holy Spirit. Yet it would be unusual for the Holy Spirit to touch him. This criterion applies to the sense of the possession—whether it is used in a negative or positive way as defined by the congregation of initiates.

Mars (14) made the distinction between "sickness possession" and "ritual possession," where the former clearly refers to behavior of the possessed that the group does not tolerate. An example of this would be a participant who attacks a member of the congregation with an axe. In the case of spirit possession occurring in church, one might imagine a shouter who becomes so frenzied that she raises her dress or even tries to take it off. Such behavior could hardly be tolerated within the confines of the church. Interestingly enough, then, in "ritual possession" the behavior of the possessed individual is limited and confined even though the possessed person no longer controls his own body. It appears that every participant in possession rituals instinctively knows what behavior is and is not sanctioned by the group. However, they all argue that an *orisha* or a saint never directs a believer to behave in a negatively oriented way unless the horse needed to be punished for some reason or other, or unless it is a case of sickness possession and the motivation is human.

One of the most striking features of possession is the amazing similarity that exists in the behavioral manifestations of those who are being ridden by a *loa* or *orisha*. Maya Deren (15) shows two photographs, taken six months apart and in different places, of participants being possessed by Ghede, one of the Haitian deities. The two people are both sitting on a chair with legs crossed, each smoking a cigarette and with their hands in their laps. This is proof that the *loa's* "character is constant and independent of that of the person in whose body he becomes manifest." The same elementary uniformity is present in the possessions of the Black church. The shouters all bring a singular originality to their movements; but on the whole, everything they do fits into a general pattern of the shout which is identifiable to the congregation of initiates. Many of them insist that they know or remember very little of what they actually did while possessed. Still, each time that possession comes, the manifestations are similar. One wonders why there is such uniformity in the physical and observable deportment of the possessed. At the same time, this is one of the criteria of possession that creates difficulties for the psychiatrist. In the case cited, the patient's behavior was recognizable as resembling that of her Puerto Rican spiritualist peers; consequently, the other criteria needed to be invoked for the establishment of some clear differentiation.

In clinical cases, the psychiatrist has to use his judgment in a comparative sense when he applies each criterion related to possession phenomena. In the case cited the patient certainly did satisfy some criteria. However, we felt that the ones she did not satisfy were important and striking enough to make us consider her an example of abnormal possession. It must also be understood that one can find examples of possessed people who contradict our criteria. The psychiatrist must learn through clinical experience to deal with these exceptions.

CONCLUSION

Hex and spirit possession are two recurring phenomena which present problems for psychiatrists attempting to treat patients who believe in spiritualism. We have tried to clarify some of the clinical issues related to these two phenomena and we have raised questions for further research.

The effects of hex beliefs on patients need to be documented further. The documentation of cases in which the hex plays a prominent role in the genesis of the psychiatric illness is particularly important. In the cases cited, there is evidence of premorbid personality characteristics which tend to diminish the effectiveness of the claim that the hex contributed directly to the appearance of mental illness. With respect to possession, the same problem exists. The literature abounds in descriptions of normal, ritual, ceremonial possession. We need to document more cases of abnormal possession so that we can test the validity of our criteria with more effectiveness. At present, we have no way of knowing which should be major and which minor criteria in the assessment of "abnormal" states of spirit possession. With these caveats in mind, we hope this paper has contributed to increasing the effectiveness of the psychiatrist's approach to the spiritualist patient.

REFERENCES

1. Lubchansky, I., Egri, G., and Stokes, J. Puerto Rican spiritualists view mental illness: The faith healer as a paraprofessional. *Amer. J. Psychiat.*, 127 (3): 312–321, 1970.
2. Fisch, S. Botanicas and spiritualism in a metropolis. *Milbank Memorial Fund Quart. Bull.*, 46: 377–388, 1968.
3. Ruiz, P., and Langrod, J. Psychiatry and folk healing: A dichotomy? *Amer. J. Psychiat.*, 133 (1): 95–97, 1976.
4. Harwood, A. The hot-cold theory of disease: Implications for treatment of Puerto Rican patients. *J. Amer. Med. Assn.* 216: 1153–1158, 1971.
5. Cannon, W.B. "Voodoo" death. *Psychosom. Med.,* 19: 182–190, 1957.
6. Richter, C.P. On the phenomenon of sudden death in animals and man. *Psychosom. Med.,* 19: 191–198, 1957.
7. Mathis, J.L. A sophisticated version of voodoo death. *Psychosom. Med.,* 26, 104–107, 1964.
8. Cappannari, S.C., Rau, B., Abram, H.S., and Buchanan, D.C. Voodoo in the general hospital; a case of hexing and regional enteritis. *J. Amer. Med. Assn.,* 232: 938–940, 1975.
9. Mathewson, M.A. Is crazy Anglo crazy Haitian? *Psychiat. Ann.,* 5 (8): 79–83, 1975.
10. Kiev, A. Spirit possession in Haiti, *Amer. J. Psychiat.,* 118: 133-138, 1961.
11. Gonzalez-Wippler, M. *Santeria.* New York: Anchor Books, 1975.
12. Mischel, W., and Mischel, F. Psychological aspects of spirit possession. *Amer. Anthropol.,* 60: 249–260, 1958.
13. Southern, E. The religious occasion. In: C. Lincoln, ed., *The Black Experience in Religion.* New York: Anchor Books, 1974, pp. 52–63.
14. Mars, L. Phenomena of "possession." *Tomorrow: World's Dig. Psychic Occult,* 3 (1): 61–73, 1954.
15. Deren, M. *Divine Horsemen: The Voodoo Gods of Haiti.* New York: Delta Books, 1972.

9

Belief and Behavior:
Cultural Factors in the Recognition and
Treatment of Mental Illness

RONALD M. WINTROB

For at least the past decade, mental health personnel and social scientists have become increasingly aware—sometimes painfully so—that the long-accepted melting-pot theory of ethnic assimilation in the United States could no longer be supported. Accumulating historical and social-scientific evidence has been pointing to another conclusion: instead of a melting pot of ethnic assimilation, America has been evolving as a country of enduring ethnic diversity, a mosaic of cultural pluralism. Within this mosaic, we are recognizing a continuity of ethnic communities, a reaffirmation of cultural heritage of values, beliefs, and behaviors. Recent events in Boston and Pine Ridge, South Dakota, have demonstrated something of the quality of fierce assertiveness of ethnic identity and what might be thought of as the boundaries of ethnicity. Observers of our social system such as Glazer and Moynihan have been led from *Beyond the Melting Pot* (1) to the view that "perhaps the hope of doing without ethnicity in a society as its subgroups assimilate to the majority group may be as utopian and questionable an enter-

103

prise as the hope of doing without social classes in a society" (2).

From the viewpoint of clinical service provided by mental health personnel, an awareness of the importance of ethnicity in determining the diagnostic significance of clinical data is becoming evident. That this level of clinical awareness has not come about easily is illustrated by Cohen's (3) observation: "During diagnosis and treatment there is a remarkable lack of direct attention given to ethnicity, race, sub-cultural identity, and bilingualism by mental health practitioners." Cohen suggests that this relative exclusion of ethnic or cultural data may be due to conscious or unconscious avoidance resulting from many thera-pists' concern not to be "discriminating" or to "show prejudice" in their treatment of the ethnically, racially, culturally, or linguistically distinct.

Recognizing that the ideal remains distant and uncertain, it is nonetheless appropriate to look back over what has been achieved during the past decade in the recognition of ethnic and cultural diversity in peoples' explanations of mental illness and how it should be treated. To this end, I shall review the folk explanations of mental illness among several ethnic minorities, as well as subcultural groups of the dominant culture in the United States. It is a focus on the *why* of illness: why people believe the misfortune of mental illness has affected *them* rather than others, and why it has affected them *at this particular time* rather than any other time. Consideration of these questions leads people almost inevitably to ask themselves: What went wrong? *What did we do wrong* that this illness has befallen us or one of our family? And from these questions, many people are led to wonder whether someone else or some other force in the universe has had a hand in their misfortune.

NATURAL VERSUS SUPERNATURAL IN THE EXPLANATION OF ILLNESS: RECOGNITION OF THE PHENOMENON

During the past 10 years there has been a steady growth in the psychiatric literature concerning folk explanation of illness. This is not to say that there was no interest in the phenomenon in earlier years; there is a long tradition in psychiatry of interest in the relation between religious beliefs and mental illness, the religious content of disordered thought, and the restorative function of religious faith in psychiatric and psychosomatic illnesses. Furthermore, there has been some tradition of cross-cultural research in psychiatry for over 40 years. Nonetheless, the focus of earlier research on the folk explanation of mental illness, and particularly on supernatural beliefs' influence on psychopathology, was directed toward "primitive" peoples in other parts of the world. More recently, a number of research reports have appeared that focus specifically on the belief systems of ethnic minorities within the United States in relation to the causes and appropriate treatment of mental illness. The two principal groups studied to date have been American blacks and the Hispanic population of the United States. Among blacks, the system of beliefs relating illness to supernatural influence is generally called rootwork (4, 5), hexing (6), or voodoo (7); less frequently it is referred to as witchcraft or hoodoo (8).

The common theme of this belief system is that personal misfortune such as mental illness may have two principal causes: natural and unnatural. Natural causes include factors such as genetic predisposition, nutritional imbalance or infection, cruel or neglectful parenting, or the chronic stresses of poverty. Unnatural causes include fate, spirit possession, or malign magic. The concept of malign magic is central, implying that mental illness may result not from the wishes or behavior of the sufferer, but from the malevolent wishes of others. It is believed that an individual who is sufficiently envious and resentful of the achievements of another may cause harm—accident, illness, even death—through appeal to intermediaries of the spirit world. Looked at from the opposite perspective, people suffering from mental illness would regard themselves as the innocent victims of cruel fate or the machinations of envious, malevolent members of their communities.

Among Mexican-Americans, a parallel set of beliefs is generally labeled *curanderismo* (9–11), while among Puerto Ricans the equivalent belief system is most often called *espiritismo* (12–14). A similar complex of beliefs called *santeria* has been described among the Cuban population of the Miami area (15). While *curanderismo*, *espiritismo*, and *santeria* share the theme of distinguishing natural from unnatural in the causes of illness and equally emphasize the "innocent victim" role of the sufferer, there is a greater emphasis on soul loss and spirit possession as the direct or proximal causes of the manifest symptoms of disorder.

In recent years there has also been a growing interest in the beliefs of subcultural groups of whites, as well as ethnic minorities in the United States, about faith healing (16, 17) and spirit possession, or mediumship (18). There has been increasing concern with the development of healing cults in the management of mental illness, especially among fundamentalist Christian sects (19, 20), but not excluding the larger and more traditionally organized Christian denominations (21).

HOW PREVALENT IS THE FOLK EXPLANATION
OF MENTAL ILLNESS?

Early reports of hexing and rootwork beliefs among blacks in the United States emphasized the rural southern tradition of these beliefs, as did reports of faith healing and possession phenomena among fundamentalist whites. Particularly striking were descriptions of glossolalia, possession, and trance possession among adherents of snake-handling fundamentalist sects in Appalachia and the rural South (22, 23). With further study, however, there has come increasing recognition that beliefs in hex and rootwork on the one hand, and faith healing and trance possession on the other, can be found among both blacks and whites, in the South and in the North, and indeed in all parts of the country. It has become clear that there is a rapid increase in the prevalence of fundamentalist religious healing phenomena, as exemplified by Pentecostal faith healing, throughout the country. It is equally clear that the folk explanation of mental illness is prevalent among Mexican-Americans in Chicago and Denver no less than in Los Angeles and Houston, and that *espiritismo* continues to be an important and widely shared belief system among Puerto Ricans in communities "on the mainland" and in Puerto Rico.

A critical question that remains unanswered is the extent to which the folk belief systems I have described are unique to particular segments of the communities in which the beliefs are found. Most of the research conducted to date has been in communities of the urban and rural poor. The few studies that have investigated the beliefs of the middle class have tended to support the assumption that the folk belief system crosses divisions of social class just as it does ethnic groups, but this assumption requires verification.

A FOCAL EXAMPLE: FOLK BELIEFS
ABOUT MENTAL ILLNESS IN CONNECTICUT

Connecticut's population of 3.3 million includes more than 200,000 blacks and close to 40,000 Puerto Ricans. Beginning in 1970, we have undertaken at the University of Connecticut a series of studies on the beliefs of these two ethnic groups concerning the causes and appropriate treatment of mental illness. Our study population has included a random sample of community residents and individuals who have received treatment for mental illness as inpatients or outpatients. We began with the questions: Does a system of folk beliefs exist, and if so, to what

extent are the beliefs of psychiatric patients represer
ethnic groups as a whole? We have found that rootwoi
blacks are well known in the community and widel
explanations of mental illness. These findings apply equ...,
under treatment for mental illness and those with no history of coi.
with mental health services (24, 25). Nearly half the patients interviewed
attributed their own illnesses to the effects of malign magic perpetrated
by a close relative or friend who often figured prominently in the
presenting symptomatology of acutely psychotic patients. Furthermore,
we encountered among our subjects many who were reluctant to discuss
rootwork or to remain near those who were discussing it because of
what we came to define as a fear of rootwork contamination: the notion
that it was not safe to discuss the spirit world because of the risk of
being victimized by it (24). Finally, our research has provided some
support, though limited in its significance by the small number of cases,
for the assumption that the folk belief system is not confined to people
of the lower levels of income and education. Nor are rootwork beliefs
held only by people who have migrated from the rural South.

Our research with the Puerto Rican population has likewise demonstrated that beliefs in *espiritismo* or spiritism are prevalent in the
community and are described similarly by patients and randomly selected
community residents. In addition to citing spiritism and witchcraft as
factors of major significance among natural causes of mental illness,
some subjects also mentioned *susto* or soul loss, and *desgaste* or fatigue
of the brain as causative factors (14, 26). We did not encounter among
Puerto Rican subjects a resistance to discussing spiritism analogous to
the "fear of rootwork contamination" shown by some black subjects.

During the past two years, we have had the opportunity to treat
a number of people, both whites and blacks, whose presenting symptomatology reflected an intense preoccupation with fundamentalist Christian beliefs. These patients have been very active participants in
faith-healing ceremonies including ritual trance, spirit possession, and
glossolalia. As a follow-up on these cases, we have recently begun
research in a rural and an urban setting on the psychotherapeutic effects
of fundamentalist ritual.

ATTITUDES TO TREATMENT: COMMUNITY HEALERS OR MENTAL HEALTH PROFESSIONALS?

Inevitably, investigation of peoples' beliefs about the causes of
mental illness leads one to question subjects about their attitudes to

treatment. It would seem to be a logical assumption that people who believe that some forms of mental illness are caused by unnatural factors, such as malign magic and spirit possession, would recommend forms of treatment to remove the spell or intrusive spirit, and that just such forms of treatment would exist in their communities. These assumptions have proven to be correct. Virtually all research that has established the existence of a folk belief system in a given community has also demonstrated the existence of a viable, well-recognized, and widely utilized network of local remedies and community healers.

Our research in Connecticut has confirmed that the more convinced the mentally ill person is that his illness has been caused by unnatural factors, the more likely it is that he will first seek the help of a community healer—rootworker, spiritist, or curer. He will do so even if his family and friends are opposed to community healers or unconvinced of the effectiveness of their treatment. In our experience, though, it is more often the case that the patient's family and friends are supportive and urge the patient to get help from local healers. In our study of the Puerto Rican population, for example, we found that 20 percent of the random sample of people we interviewed in the community felt that the most appropriate form of treatment for mental illness was confinement at a mental hospital; 40 percent preferred treatment by a doctor—by which they generally meant a family doctor; and 40 percent recommended treatment by a spiritist. Among Puerto Ricans under treatment at a mental health center, 40 percent had been advised by their family and friends to consult a doctor for help, while 45 percent had been recommended to a community healer. Asked about the effectiveness of spiritist treatment, 70 percent of community subjects and 75 percent of mental health center patients gave favorable comments (26).

Several investigators have contended, and Torrey (27) most forcefully, that the similarities in treatment provided by indigenous healers and by psychiatrists outweigh the differences. Torrey has marshalled considerable evidence in support of this thesis. But our research in Connecticut leads us to emphasize certain crucial differences. First, our subjects, whether black, Puerto Rican, or white, clearly differentiate between mental disorders on the basis of their assumed causes—whether natural or unnatural. Second, treatment by community healers generally is believed to be effective and the treatment of choice for unnatural forms of illness, whereas hospitals and doctors are thought to be the treatment of first appeal for natural illnesses. Third, hospitals and doctors are regarded as effective providers of symptomatic relief for manifest symptomatology, or what might be considered the proximal cause of distress—such as the pain of a fracture, or auditory hallucinations. But relief from the distal or underlying cause, from the questioning about why the illness occurred, leads many patients to consider the factors of malign intervention or spirit possession—and relief from these kinds of disorders can only be provided by community healers knowledgeable about such types of illness. Only they can act as intermediaries with the spirit world and offer hope for cure. For these reasons, it seems to us that the distinguishing differences between community healers and mental health professionals should be kept clearly in mind. Viewed from this perspective, the question of who is *more* effective, community healer or mental health professional, no longer takes on the dimensions of a clarion call to defend one's territory, but recognizes the integrity and effectiveness of both groups of helpers. The operative question becomes: Who is more effective to treat what condition under what psychocultural circumstances?

CONCLUSION: DOES CULTURE COUNT?

Looking back on developments in cultural psychiatry over the past decade, there has certainly been an encouraging burgeoning of literature in the area of folk beliefs concerning the causes and treatment of mental illness. The growth of this body of literature has coincided with a broader perspective in the social sciences that has affirmed the validity and enduring vitality of the concept of cultural diversity in the social fabric of American life. Medical practitioners in general, and psychiatrists in particular, have become participants in the community, not only as observers and researchers, but as planners and providers of care for large segments of population—sometimes to the dismay, encouragement, and despair of planners, researchers, and community inhabitants alike (28, 29). However much the turbulent events in the social history of the United States during the past decade have contributed to the increased recognition of the validity of cultural pluralism, cultural psychiatry has certainly benefited. The study of folk beliefs in illness has advanced considerably. The disciplines of medical anthropology and cultural psychiatry appear to be coming of age as a more receptive audience has emerged in medicine and the social sciences. That audience recognizes that ethnic differences are reflected in differences in peoples' assessment of threats to their psychosocial security, in their interpretation of the symbolic meaning of those threats, and in their adaptive strategies to cope with threats to their security. There is a corollary recognition of the validity of alternative healing systems and the logic of treatment by community healers, no less than by professional healers. If this process continues, it should augur well for the health of the community and the discipline of psychiatry.

Presented at the Symposium on Current Issues in Transcultural Research, American Psychiatric Association meeting, Miami Beach, May 1976.

REFERENCES

1. Glazer, N., and Moynihan, D.P. *Beyond the Melting Pot*. Cambridge: MIT Press, 1970.
2. Glazer, N., and Moynihan, D.P. (eds.). *Ethnicity, Theory, and Experience*. Cambridge: Harvard University Press, 1975.
3. Cohen, R.E. Borderline conditions: A transcultural approach. *Psychiat. Ann.*, 4: 7–23, 1974.
4. Snow, L.F. Folk medical beliefs and their implications for care of patients. *Ann. Int. Med.*, 81: 82–96, 1974.
5. Tinling, D.C. Voodoo, rootwork, and medicine. *Psychosom. Med.*, 29: 483–491, 1967.
6. Snell, J.E. Hypnosis in the treatment of the hexed patient. *Amer. J. Psychiat.*, 124: 311–316, 1970.
7. Jordan, W.C. Voodoo medicine. In: *Textbook of Black-Related Diseases*, ed. R.A. Williams. New York: McGraw-Hill, 1975.
8. Maduro, R.J. Voodoo possession in San Francisco: Notes on therapeutic aspects of regression. *Ethos*, 3: 425–445, 1975.
9. Kiev, A. *Curanderismo: Mexican-American Folk Psychiatry*. New York: Free Press, 1968.
10. Clark, M. *Health in the Mexican-American Culture*, 2nd ed. Berkeley: University of California Press, 1970.
11. Edgerton, R.B., and Karno, M. Mexican-American bilingualism in perception of mental illness. *Arch. Gen. Psychiat.*, 24: 286–290, 1971.
12. Lubchansky, I., Egri, G., and Stokes, J. Puerto Rican spiritualists view mental illness: The faith healer as a paraprofessional. *Amer. J. Psychiat.*, 127: 88–97, 1970.
13. Abad, V., Ramos, J., and Boyce, E. A model for delivery of mental health services to Spanish-speaking minorities. *Amer. J. Orthopsychiat.*, 44: 584–595, 1974.
14. Gaviria, M., and Wintrob, R.M. Supernatural influence in psychopathology: Puerto Rican folk beliefs about mental illness. *Can. Psychiat. Assn. J.* 21: 361–369, 1976.
15. Sandoval, M.C., and Tozo, L. An emergent Cuban community. *Psychiat. Ann.*, 5: 324–332, 1975.
16. Pattison, E.M., Lapins, W., and Doerr, H. Faith healing: A study of personality and function. *J. Nerv. Ment. Dis.*, 157: 397–409, 1973.
17. Macklin, J. Belief, ritual, and healing: New England spiritualism and

Mexican-American spiritualism compared. In: *Religious Movements in Contemporary America,* ed. I. Zaretsky and M. Leone. Princeton: Princeton University Press, 1974.

18. Lauer, R. A medium for mental health. In: *Religious Movements in Contemporary America,* ed. I. Zaretsky and M. Leone. Princeton: Princeton University Press, 1974.

19. Garrison, V. Sectarianism and psychosocial adjustment: A controlled comparison of Puerto Rican Pentecostals and Catholics. In: *Religious Movements in Contemporary America,* ed. I. Zaretsky and M. Leone. Princeton: Princeton University Press, 1974.

20. Pattison, E.M. Ideological support for the marginal middle class: Faith healing and glossolalia. In: *Religious Movements in Contemporary America,* ed. I. Zaretsky and M. Leone. Princeton: Princeton University Press, 1974.

21. Frank, J. Religious healing. In: *Persuasion and Healing,* 2nd ed. Baltimore: Johns Hopkins University Press, 1973.

22. Kane, S. Ritual possession in a southern Appalachian religious sect. *J. Amer. Folklore,* 87: 293–302, 1975.

23. Tellegen, A., Gerrard, N.L., Gerrard, L.B., and Butcher, J.N. Personality characteristics of members of a serpent-handling religious cult. In: *MMPI: Research Developments and Clinical Applications,* ed. J.N. Butcher. New York: McGraw-Hill, 1969.

24. Wintrob, R.M., and Fox, R.A. Rootwork beliefs and psychiatric disorder among blacks in a northern U.S. city. Presented at the Fifth World Congress of Psychiatry, Mexico City, December, 1971.

25. Wintrob, R.M. The influence of others: Witchcraft and rootwok as explanations of behavior disturbances. *J. Nerv. Ment. Dis.,* 156: 318–326, 1973.

26. Wintrob, R.M., and Gaviria, M. Psychiatry in the multi-ethnic community: Psychiatrist or spirit healer in the treatment of mental illness. Presented at the 14th International Meeting of Psychiatric Outpatient Centers of America, June, 1976.

27. Torrey, E.F. *The Mind Game: Witchdoctors and Psychiatrists.* New York: Emerson Hall, 1972.

28. Lathem, W. Community medicine: Success or failure? *New Eng. J. Med.,* 295: 18–23, 1976.

29. Langsley, D.G., and Barter, J.T. Community alternatives to hospital treatment. *Psychiat. Ann.,* 5: 163–206, 1975.

10

Chinese-Speaking Vietnamese Refugees in Los Angeles: A Preliminary Investigation

JOE YAMAMOTO
JULIA LAM
DESMOND FUNG
FRANK TAN
MAMORU IGA

For centuries invaders have occupied Vietnam—first the recurrent Chinese Mandarins, followed more recently by the French, and during World War II, the Japanese. The United States was the last invader. Vietnam is a hot, humid country with rich soil and access to the ocean.

With the decision to withdraw American troops in the spring of 1975, a refugee problem immediately developed. Over one hundred thousand refugees were evacuated by the American forces or escaped by ship. They were sent to Guam and to other centers in the U.S., including Camp Pendleton, California. There they lived in tents, suffered from the cool weather, and attempted to adjust to their new and foreign environment.

We visited Camp Pendleton and were impressed with the rapid and efficient work of those engaged in resettling. The refugees are still not permanently resettled and we do not minimize the problems and difficulties. The point is that despite the urgency and the problems of the economic recession, a very large group of refugees have found

113

sponsors and attempts were made to find jobs, though many remain unemployed.

The refugees have been uprooted from their homes and their homeland, their extended kinship relations have been disrupted, and they have lost their jobs, professional status, financial security, language facility, accustomed climate, etc. (1, 2). Because of these major psychosocial transitions and the real problems (such as language, being Asian, and living in a new culture), we hypothesized that they would be under stress and therefore at risk medically and psychiatrically (3). We therefore proposed a field study of the Vietnam refugees.

Our initial plan was to request that refugees complete questionnaires as they were seen for social services and assistance for resettlement problems. However, it was soon clear that the refugees would not comply (even though the questionnaires were available in English, Vietnamese, and Chinese).

Since 10 to 20 percent of the Vietnamese refugees were Chinese, it was decided to interview them in their homes. This decision was made because of the lack of compliance in the original group and because three of the investigators were bilingual and could interview these refugees in Chinese (Cantonese).

METHODS

We had a list of 17 refugee families' names and addresses. An attempt was made to contact all of the families. Two families were never home when the interviewers tried to see them and one family had moved away. Thus, 14 families were seen in their homes. Our original intention was to interview the head of the household and/or other adult refugees, using a detailed demographic questionnaire form printed in English, Vietnamese, and Chinese. In addition, we asked each participating adult to complete the modified Berger Self-Conception Scale, the Spielberger State Trait Anxiety Scale, and the Zung Self-Rating Depression Scale. The tests were translated by us when necessary into Vietnamese and Chinese so that all data collected were available in all three languages. The Zung Scale was already available in Chinese. There was a Vietnamese version of the Spielberger Scale which we modified. Completed questionnaires were obtained after much encouragement and persistence. Although the final results have not been tabulated, we have some preliminary figures. As with all field research, we do not have every form completed by every possible adult. Some were illiterate and would not complete the forms.

We found that half, seven out of the 14, had missing family members (4, 5). For example, one family had arrived without the eldest son and his family. Another family had been unable to bring two sons from Vietnam. A third family had left four children of whom two were in Vietnam and two in Taiwan. Still another family headed by a widower had left two children who somehow were lost in the rush to escape Vietnam. Another family left the wife and five children in Taiwan. A young boy, age 14, and his oldest sister, age 16, were sent to Los Angeles to await their parents and siblings who are in Taiwan. Another woman came to the U. S. with her daughter and awaits her husband and five other children who are in Taiwan. This is an example of what we felt would be a crucial variable, that is, the absence of family members, especially those who were left in Vietnam. Those in Taiwan could more surely immigrate later.

We examined occupational data to determine whether joblessness contributed to the refugees' feelings of anxiety and depression. In our sample, there were no heads of the household who spoke English. This limited work opportunities. In reference to vocational adjustment, those who came from working-class backgrounds tended to be better adjusted. The jobs mentioned by those employed were menial and physical, e.g., waitressing or cleaning poultry.

In our discussions with the refugees it was surprising how hospitable and open they were. We were welcomed and they were appreciative of our interests. We advised the refugees about how to obtain medical services—how to get a Med-i-Cal Card (California Medicaid)—counseled them about how to arrange for the immigration of their relatives, and gave them other practical pointers.

Families were visited more than once. They commented on their feeling disappointed in the local community. One refugee, for example, said, "We were much more hospitable to refugees who came to Vietnam." This was a very frequent complaint.

One of the objectives of our field study was to determine whether some immigrants needed psychiatric treatment, such as crisis-intervention therapy, or other psychological services. One woman was moderately depressed and was offered an appointment for psychiatric help, but she refused. Thus far, we have not treated any refugees for depression or other emotional symptoms.

PRELIMINARY RESULTS

There were 98 members of the 14 families. Each family thus had an average of seven members. We found that only 73 of the 98 family members had actually been able to leave Vietnam. Of the 25 left in

Asia, there were seven still in Vietnam and 18 in Taiwan. We wondered if the difference between the permitted immigration from Taiwan and the uncertainties of the situation in Vietnam would add to the stress.

In our field interviews of the families, we used the Walter Reed Mental Status Schedule as a starting point and as a guideline in conducting various aspects of the mental status examination. Together with checks on the modified form, each family had a global clinical evaluation. In reviewing the records, it was found that there were four families where there seemed to be significant depression, the evaluation being of "moderate depression." There were six families who were felt to be slightly depressed and four where there was no evidence of depression.

In the interviews in the refugees' homes, all were hospitable and expressed appreciation to the United States Government. Their adaptational problems were determined largely by the different priorities of the sponsors and refugees. The most frequently mentioned problem was that the Christian sponsors insisted the Vietnamese attend church despite the fact that they were Buddhist. The local Asian community was seen as less hospitable. None of the refugees interviewed spoke English, although many said they were learning. This was an important problem. In Los Angeles, none had automobiles and this was another problem. We found that those who were clinically rated as being depressed scored higher on the Zung Scale. Table 1 shows that the moderately depressed averaged 52, slightly depressed 53, and those without depression averaged 46. Similarly, the average scores on the Spielberger Scale for the moderately depressed families were 43, slightly depressed families, 48; and the families not depressed at all, 41.

Because Asians value work, we felt jobs would be very important. We examined those families who were moderately depressed and the table shows that we found that all four families had an unemployed head of the household. Of the six families with slight depression, three had unemployed heads of the household. Of the four families who showed no clinical depression, none were unemployed, though one widower was retired. Comparing the depressed and not depressed group, we found a difference significant at the .05 level.

In order to evaluate the effects of being separated from members of the nuclear family, we examined those instances where family members were absent. Seven out of the 14 families had someone still in Asia. However, we found that these families were scattered among those who seemed to be depressed and those who were not. Among the moderately depressed families, one family had children in Vietnam and another had relatives in Taiwan. Of the slightly depressed families, there was one family with children in both Vietnam and Taiwan, an-

Table 1
Depression Ratings

		Average Zung Score	Average Spielberger Score	Unemployed Head of Household
Moderately Depressed	(4 Families)	52	43	4/4
Slightly Depressed	(6 Families)	53	48	3/6
Not Depressed	(4 Families)	46	41	0/4

	Employed	Unemployed
Depressed	3	7
Not Depressed	4	0

p = .05 using Fisher's Exact Test

other family with children in Vietnam and still another with relatives in Taiwan. Of those families with no apparent clinical depression, one had children still in Vietnam and another family had parents and siblings in Taiwan. Thus, exactly half of the refugee families in each clinical category had relatives still in Asia.

DISCUSSION

The evacuation of the Vietnamese refugees in the spring of 1975 and their resettlement in a new culture suggested there would be increased stress, anxiety, and depression. We interviewed 14 families of Chinese-speaking refugees from Vietnam. There were many variables we felt would contribute towards successful adaptation and many others that would impede adaptation. Most of the families shared common problems related to language, sponsorship, disappointment in the local Asian community, and concern about employment. Seven out of the 14 families still had children, siblings, and/or parents either in Vietnam or Taiwan. Though we had speculated that those with relatives in Vietnam would be more distressed, our methods did not reveal significant differences. The most impressive finding was the pattern of clinical depression as related to employment. We found that there were four families with moderate depression, six with slight depression, and four without apparent depression. The average scores on the Zung Self-Rating Depression Scale and the Spielberger Anxiety Scale tended to bear out the clinical impressions.

Of the four families that were moderately depressed, all had an unemployed head of the household, three of the six slightly depressed families were similarly unemployed, while none of the four families without depression had an unemployed head of the household. This was a significant difference.

Our findings suggest that jobs for Vietnamese refugees should have top priority. In addition, they need English lessons and orientation to American ways. While a few may need psychiatric treatment, they will reject such an offer because of cultural bias against psychiatry.

Presented at the Annual Meeting of the American Psychiatric Association, May, 1976, Miami Beach, Florida.

REFERENCES

1. Chu, H-M. Migration and mental disorders in Taiwan. In: *Transcultural Research in Mental Health*, ed. W.P. Lebra. Honolulu: University Press of Hawaii, 1972, pp. 295–325.
2. Murphy, H.B.M. Psychiatric concomitants of fusion in plural societies.
3. Holmes, H., and Masuda, M. Life change and illness susceptibility. In: *Stressful Life Events*, ed. B.S. Dohrenwend and B.P. Dohrenwend. New York: Wiley, 1973, pp. 45–73.
4. Forrest, D.V. Vietnamese maturation: The lost land of bliss. *Psychiatry*, 34: 111–139, 1971.
5. Tran-Ming Tung. The family and the management of mental health problems in Vietnam. In: *Transultural Research in Mental Health*, ed. W.P. Lebra. Honolulu: University Press of Hawaii, 1972, Chap. 7.

Part III
CROSS-CULTURAL RESEARCH BY AMERICAN PSYCHIATRISTS OUTSIDE OF NORTH AMERICA

Introduction

JOSEPH WESTERMEYER

Why leave North America to study psychiatric disorder? This is an important question, one well worth asking before undertaking research elsewhere, since research in foreign countries is expensive and time-consuming. Moreover, it often does not relate directly to psychiatric problems here in our own country. In considering such research, the investigator might first ask, "What useful projects might I undertake in this or that exotic place I would like to visit?" A more useful beginning question would be, "Can this research question be adequately answered in my own society?" If it can, the priority for cross-cultural research dwindles.

There are, however, problems that can be best investigated by cross-cultural research in cultures significantly different from our own. These include topics such as the following: (1) sociocultural influences determining the incidence, prevalence, or form of psychiatric disorder; (2) the social role of psychiatric practitioners in various societies; (3) the effectiveness of specific psychiatric treatment modalities in different cultural settings; (4) psychiatric disorders that occur infrequently in our society, but more commonly in other societes (e.g., the so-called culture-bound syndromes, including amok, latah); (5) assessment of possible sociocultural causes for the relative infrequency of certain problems in some societies (e.g., low rates of suicide, essential hypertension, alcoholism).

The cross-cultural approach offers certain inherent methodologic advantages. It can overcome ethnocentric bias in the investigator; we often see cultural issues more clearly in other societies, while remaining blissfully unaware of mores and values within our own group. In addition, biases and expectations on the part of the subject may diminish as the psychiatrist-researcher enters other, more remote societies. (For example, I found it considerably easier to enter the social milieu of tribal societies in Asia than the social milieu of tribal societies in Minnesota.) And, in order to test certain sociocultural hypotheses, one often needs findings from a variety of societies in order to show whether the theory can be validated or whether another theory is needed.

In addition to the usual logistics problems of any research, special problems attend carefully done cross-cultural research. The investigator must spend months, and usually years, in learning and adapting to the indigenous culture. This usually involves learning another language and/or learning the nuances of conducting a mental status examination through a translator. Assumption of a social role that can be understood and accepted by the subjects is a critical step. In most cases there are special difficulties in obtaining a random or even a representative sample.

Two current problems for such studies should be mentioned. The first is the need for careful ethnographic reading before collecting data, careful research methodology, linguistic training for the psychiatrist-researcher and/or training of translators, and immersion into a culture for at least one or two years. This demands time, commitment, and training. Secondly there is a dearth of available resources. Psychiatrists working in this field must usually fund their own research or seek new employment in the region where they wish to undertake their research. This latter constraint has limited our field to a few highly motivated psychiatrists willing to abandon more popular and lucrative pursuits. While this status quo may have utility in a relatively new field, it severely limits the work that can be accomplished and discourages bright young research psychiatrists who might otherwise be attracted to this field.

Dr. Beiser raises two important issues that are increasingly discussed by those of us doing cross-cultural research. First, what are the ethical aspects in the project under consideration? And second, what are the researcher's obligations to the population being studied? Unlike those of us who have reflected on these dilemmas privately, Dr. Beiser publicly shares his observations, experiences, and reservations. He also indicates that simple answers to these problems are not in the offing. Research ethics in a tribal society are *not* the same as in an American metropolis. In tribal settings, many decisions are made on a community rather than on an individual basis. Or, as Dr. Beiser points out, a verbal willingness to cooperate with research activities can readily be negated by the subject's behavior ("I have to go and visit my cousin"). The first step toward solving difficult problems is to frame critical questions. Dr. Beiser has assisted those of us interested in cross-cultural research by posing these queries.

Art has been used as a diagnostic tool and as a therapeutic modality in the Occidental world for decades. Dr. Billig's work in recent years has established the utility of art as a cross-cultural research instrument. Much of his work has been among schizophrenic patients. He has demonstrated that, while artistic content varies from one culture to another, the step-by-step impact of thought disorder on artistic form is quite uniform depending upon the severity of clinical impairment. Dr. Billig's work has demonstrated the uniformity of the schizophrenic process regardless of the individual's literacy, occupation, or sociocultural milieu.

Dr. Burton-Bradley's paper demonstrates the continued utility of the intensive case study in understanding psychiatric disorder. The influences of biological, psychological, and sociocultural factors are all evident in his paper. The sociocultural elements, in this case specific to Papua New Guinea, include cannibalism, cargo cultism, and the influences of Occidental technology and Christian missionaries. In addition, Dr. Burton-Bradley contributes a new concept to anthropology: cargo thinking. This term refers to grandiose, passive, magical expectation in a setting of sudden, momentous technologic and cultural change. Finally, his paper raises major ethical and political issues regarding the influence of proselytizing religions, transplanted whole cloth out of Occidental society into vastly different culture areas.

In her data from Surinam, Dr. Houston presents a folk classification of psychiatric disorder among two black tribes. Of special interest is the fact that these people are descendants of African slaves who fought for and obtained their freedom in the mid-eighteenth century. Thus, they have preserved many cultural forms shared by black people brought to North and South America; however, in most other instances these mores have been diluted by contact with Indian, Latin, and Euro-American cultures. These data provide an important link between folk psychiatry from tribal Africa and folk psychiatry as encountered in the Caribbean, Latin America, and the United States. Through Dr. Houston's vivid descriptions, one can envision linkages between Caribbean voodoo, American rootwork, and the rich, varied folk psychiatries of Africa.

Dr. Westermeyer's paper comprises a distillation of field studies on opium addiction conducted over a 10-year period. By providing another cultural "case" of narcotic addiction, these data have aided in assessing what aspects of heroin addiction in the United States can be attributed to heroin and what aspects to American social forms. The study further suggests that treatment for narcotic addiction is welcomed by Asian addicts and their families. Given favorable conditions during the post-treatment period, treatment can be as efficacious as treatment for alcoholism among middle-class Americans.

11

Ethics in Cross-Cultural Research

MORTON BEISER

In 1971, a group of colleagues from the University of Dakar and I conducted a survey of urban migrants and traditional villagers in Senegal. We were studying the effects of rapid social change on the mental and physical health of the Serer tribe, who, after a long period of isolation from the modern world, were now becoming caught up in it.

In 1975, I went back to Senegal to find out what had happened to the original sample of 504 people. Much to my delight, Thiere D., a Serer who had participated in the 1971 study, agreed to rejoin me for this phase of the work. On the day we were to set out from Dakar for the Sine-Saloum, home of the Serer for the past 800 years, I found Thiere uncharacteristically reticent and withdrawn. My urgings to tell me what was on his mind at first met no response, but finally he replied, "I must speak to you now as a friend. Before we go back to the villages, you should be ready to answer a question. The people will ask you why, after your study, so many of them became sick. I ask that question myself."

Research for this chapter was carried out while the author was a member of the Harvard Program in Social Psychiatry and a Macy Foundation Faculty Scholar 1974–75.

I had no answer. The best I could do was share with Thiere the surprise and concern he had made me feel. Fortunately, Thiere's friendship for me and his influence within the tribe sheltered me from what could have been a difficult situation; he made it possible for me to go back to talk to people and find out more about how our study had affected their lives.

That experience raised many new questions which, in an attempt to construct guides to my perplexity, I reduced to several overall themes. These included:

1. Can we go beyond broad generalizations such as, "one needs to understand a culture in order to work in it," and begin to specify some of the problems of doing research in foreign cultures?

2. What does consent mean in a culture such as that of the Serer?

3. Can research such as ours do harm?

4. What are the responsibilities of a research team to the population with which they do work?

This paper constitutes a preliminary attempt to come to terms with these issues.

BACKGROUND, SETTING, AND CONDUCT OF STUDY

Senegal, a nation of 4,000,000 people, gained political independence from France in 1960. It is a land peopled by diverse ethnic groups among whom the Serer, numbering about 400,000, are the most traditional. Thirty-five thousand Serer live in the Sine-Saloum, a region which, because it is geographically isolated and because it possesses few natural resources, has been of little interest to the outside world. The Serer, who have lived in the Sine for at least 800 years, have maintained a stability so remarkable that a French anthropologist (1) was moved to call the region a "museum of Serer culture."

During the past 20 years, however, even the Sine has changed. Population increases, overuse of the land leading to exhaustion, and a recent severe drought in West Africa have combined to create a situation in which the agriculturally based economy can no longer support the Serer in their traditional way of life. As in many other developing countries, people try to solve their difficulties by migrating to the cities.

The largest city in Senegal, one which attracts many Serer, is Dakar. It is also the capital, the center of industry and commerce, the site of a highly respected university, and one of the most cosmopolitan cities in Africa.

Our study took place in these two areas—the Sine-Saloum and

Dakar. We wanted to know what happened to urban migrants who, forced into contact with Europeans and other Africans they had never met before, exposed to twentieth-century technology, and facing an urban way of life for the first time, were trying to cope. The question possessed more than academic interest; the World Health Organization and the Ministry of Health for Senegal wanted some of the answers such a study would provide in order to help plan for the mental health needs of the Senegalese people. Three institutions provided support and encouragement for our study—the university, government, and the World Health Organization.

The first research problem we faced was how to construct a representative sample of urban and rural Serer. We were fortunate in that Niakhar, the region of the Sine-Saloum we had selected as our rural base, had been studied several years before by the Office de Recherche Scientifique et Technique Outre-Mer (ORSTOM). This agency, a research office of the French government, had collected data about economic conditions, religious preferences, and physical characteristics in each of the 65 villages in our study area. ORSTOM generously shared these data with us.

Using factor analysis, we reduced these data to three factors: (1) economic progressiveness, (2) exposure to the outside world, and (3) population stability. We divided all the factor scores into high, medium, or low for the first factor and high or low for the remaining two. This created a possibility for 12 different categories ($3 \times 2 \times 2$) and each village could be assigned to one of the 12 categories based on its profile of scores. For example, villages high on economic progressiveness, high on openness to the outside world, and high on population stability made up Category I, villages high on economic progressiveness, high on openness to the outside world, but low on population stability made up Category II, and so forth. By random sampling we selected one village from each category and then conducted a census of all adult residents. The final step was to select a probability sample of 25 adults from each village, giving us a total sample of 300.

In the city, we relied on our Serer informants to identify the four major areas where the Serer from the Sine-Saloum came to live and we then conducted a total enumeration of all Serer in these areas. Again, we chose a sample of these adult Serer on a probability basis. (Those with a specific interest in our sampling may wish to peruse [2] and [3], where the method is discussed in greater depth.)

We faced another problem common to all research workers in cross-cultural psychiatry. How does one define and measure psychiatric disorder in a culture radically different from one's own and in an area where endemic physical illnesses may be confused with emotional upsets?

Our attempts to deal with these very complex and very important issues must be presented in a detailed fashion elsewhere. However, a brief description of our methods provides some necessary context for later sections of this report. We approached the first question by constructing a lexicon of Serer disease terms and coming to an understanding of what disease means in this context by examining a number of Serer-defined "patients." This gave us some understanding of the translatability of our psychiatric system in Serer terms and vice versa, and also supplied us with a listing of symptoms by which the Serer expressed their discomforts. The symptom list was incorporated into a questionnaire which we administered, in Serer, to all the people in our samples. In order to deal with the confounding effects of physical illness, we performed physical examinations, supplemented by blood and urine analyses and radiograms (for further detail, see [2, 4, 5]).

UNDERSTANDING THE CULTURE: WHAT DOES THIS MEAN?

I have detailed some of our procedures, hoping to illustrate that, in spite of inevitable imperfections, they conform to standards of scientific rigor appropriate to this kind of work. In other words, within a Western-oriented medicoscientific framework, this study makes sense.

We realized, of course, that we were working with our feet in two camps—the subculture of Western science and the society of the Serer. In spite of this insight, we failed to anticipate how some of the ideas and methods *we* took for granted would create difficulties in the Sine-Saloum.

Explaining to people why and how they have been chosen to be members of our sample provides a good example. Most people who are not statisticians have some difficulty grasping concepts like probability and representative samplings. However, in the Western world, the idea of chance, which is related to these concepts, is at least understood and accepted. To a Serer, chance has no meaning. In his culture everything—sickness, health, misfortune, or a good yield from his field—depends upon the will of the gods or the intercession of guardian spirits.

We knew this and tried to introduce our ideas about chance to the Serer by playing games such as dice throwing with them. How naïve we were. If a Serer won a throw of the die, it was because a guardian spirit had chosen to be good to him, not because of the thing we called chance.

Our sampling method created another, more serious problem. By the very nature of the procedure, we singled out individuals for study, something that is antithetical to the Serer way of life. Individuality and achievement, prominent values for us, mean little to the Serer. The individual belongs to a social group in a very profound sense; the family, the clan, the village form his identity and he does not divorce himself from it. When I have described our Serer respondents' reticence about being interviewed to some of my Western colleagues, I have been struck by how often these colleagues respond with a statement such as, "Well naturally, people object to an invasion of their privacy," or, "Even if you have reassured people that they are being picked at random, they still suspect that you have a reason—that maybe they are mentally ill, or that others will think of them as ill afterwards."

I do not believe either interpretation to be valid. First of all, the Serer do not think of privacy as we do. One always finds Serer in groups; someone who wishes to be alone will be considered ill or at least very odd. One of the first things I, as a research worker living among the Serer, had to learn was that their insistence that someone always be with me, constituted an act of kindness, not an invasion of my privacy. Nor do I think that the informants were too concerned about being labeled as ill because they had been chosen for our study. Once again, Serer notions about illness, especially mental illness, are very different from our own. According to their beliefs, most of these illnesses are caused by spirits or by witchcraft. Since people who become ill are less at fault than they are unfortunate, and since they can be expected to recover, mental sickness does not carry with it the stigma it does in our culture.

In order to understand what disturbed the Serer about our singling out individuals, I have found it helpful to refer to the Old Testament text in which an individual is enjoined not to extend the roof of his tent beyond those of his neighbors'. Our modern society is competitive, but the society which gave rise to that biblical injunction was, as Serer society still is, interdependent. The Sine-Saloum, a dry, barren, harsh land, provides a home in which no one person or small group could hope to survive; this is why the word in Serer that comes closest to our notion of "crazy" translates literally as "he who would walk alone in the bush." Choosing persons as individuals to take part in our study constituted a threat to this interdependence and undoubtedly mobilized some resistance.

The foregoing remarks apply to our rural group, the Serer of the Sine. It is remarkable how much the traditional culture persists in Dakar; nevertheless there are changes. A national lottery has familiarized at least some people with the notion of chance and the more competitive, less communal way of life in a city makes it easier to deal with sampling on an individual basis.

The conduct of the examinations themselves, particularly the physical examinations, created difficulties we did not appreciate until it was too late to rectify the situation. Part of the difficulty again stems from cultural misunderstandings. To the outside eye, the Serer are much more casual about dress than Westerners. Children often run naked in the villages, women are barebreasted and nurse the children openly, and men wear skimpy clothing in hot weather. The examining physicians, seeing greater latitude than they were accustomed to, made the mistake of assuming that there were *no* rules governing personal modesty or appropriate behavior between the sexes. Only after the studies had been completed did we begin to hear complaints about having male doctors examining females, or about examinations of adults being conducted in the presence of children. Subjects were sometimes asked, in the presence of children, to produce a urine specimen—something apparently not openly discussed in polite Serer society.

WHAT DOES CONSENT MEAN IN THE SERER CULTURE?

In the Western world, we have become increasingly concerned with protecting the human rights of research subjects. The Nuremberg Code (6), which provides the basis for much of our thinking about research ethics, takes up the issue of informed consent as its first principle:

> The voluntary consent of the human subject is essential. This means that the person involved should have the legal capacity to give consent; should be so situated as to be able to exercise free power of choice, without the intervention of any element of force, fraud, deceit, duress, overreaching or other ulterior form of restraint or coercion; and should have sufficient knowledge and comprehension of the elements of the subject matter involved as to enable him to make an understanding and enlightened decision.

Surely there can be no quarrel with the spirit of this statement. However, this and most other formulations about consent address themselves to the individual for, in our system of values, an individual must have ultimate freedom of choice. In the Sine-Saloum, group consensus interacts with individual acquiescence in interesting ways. In order to obtain permission to work in a village, we found we had to first meet with the village chief and allow him to form an opinion about us and to exchange gifts with us. If he approved of us, he then arranged a meeting which was attended by many other people, notably the compound and family chiefs. During these meetings, we described the aims of the study, detailed the procedures, and answered questions. Only once a unanimous decision was reached, and only if it was unanimously favorable, could we proceed further. (One of the villages did refuse to cooperate with us and we reluctantly dropped it from our sample of 12.)

Following North American research guidelines (7), we talked with the village authorities about our concern to assure individual voluntary participation; we stressed that we did not wish people to feel coerced into taking part in the study and that they must feel free to withdraw from the project if they should desire to do so. The reaction ranged from puzzlement to indignation. If the village authority gave his permission, we were told, we could and should expect complete cooperation.

It proved to be true that, once we had obtained consensus at the village level, we never encountered an outright refusal from an individual. In some villages, we obtained virtually 100 percent cooperation. In others, however, we encountered difficulties which we later came to recognize as passive forms of resistance to our study—people failing to show up for appointments, confusion about schedules, people suddenly having to be away from a village when they were supposed to be having an examination, and so forth.

In the villages where these problems were particularly prominent, we were able, in time, to identify some reasons. In several of the villages, the consent of the chief was sometimes motivated by politeness rather than conviction. A Serer will rarely say no to people whom he considers to be his friends but, if he holds a position of influence, he will find ways to communicate his reluctance to the village and the behavior of the people will follow suit. In one village in which we worked, the situation was quite different. The chief was cooperative, but his authority was under question. Naturally, since we followed our usual procedure of working first with and through him, we set ourselves up to be opposed by rival community factions. It is interesting that, under these circumstances, resistance was a result of group processes, not individual idiosyncratic decisions.

WHAT ARE THE RESPONSIBILITIES OF RESEARCH WORKERS?

Research people are notorious for asking much of their subjects and giving little in return. During our survey, we were very careful not to make any verbal promises we thought we could not honor. In particular, we stressed the idea that the study would not produce any immediate benefits but that the results would be used for long-range planning. And yet, a study like this at the very least arouses expectations and may in fact imply a promise which is ultimately violated.

How does one respond, for example, to a subject who asks, "It has been 30 years since we saw a doctor; today there are 30 in our village. How does this happen? We are ill; why will they not help us tomorrow as they are willing to, today?"

The villagers simply could not understand why we were studying healthy people when so many of them were sick and in need of attention. Even our efforts to examine and treat the sick while our medical teams were in the village provided a negligible contribution to people's well-being. After our teams left the village, people fell ill, became infirm and died, just as they always had.

And so we return to Thiere's question. If we did no good for the villagers, did we in fact do harm? He claimed that more people were complaining about illness in the villages after the survey than before, and that some people were blaming the study for their illnesses. For example, they felt that our taking blood samples had weakened some people and made them more vulnerable to illness.

Did the examinations make people ill? In a certain sense I think not. In the villages I revisited, I talked with people who had participated in the study and felt that they were now sick. The symptoms they described to me—whether fatigue, weakness, anxiousness, feelings of hopelessness and despair—were symptoms these same respondents had suffered long before our study. The symptoms were not new. What was new was the people's willingness to call these things "sickness."

How did this happen? Without any doubt, the answer to this is complex and requires extensive study. I am, however, prepared to offer a partial explanation. Before our survey, the Serer experienced symptoms, but they accepted them as inevitable or as character traits—certainly not as illness. The difference is crucial. An illness is a condition we can usually do something about; if we cannot cure an illness, we can at least name it and predict what will happen to someone who has it. Naming, predicting, and curing—in these ways, we achieve a measure of control. Fate and character, on the other hand, are beyond control. I suggest that our survey opened up a whole new way of thinking about weakness, tiredness, anxiousness, and hopelessness. We asked about these things in the context of a medical study, which suggested that they were symptoms—and if they were symptoms, then the "illness" underlying them could be cured. I have reported elsewhere (8) that, although the Serer possess concepts corresponding to our own about major mental disorders such as psychosis and epilepsy, they have no words or categories similar to our term "neurotic disorder." They do, however, experience the full range of symptoms we think of as falling within this category. I suggest that our own ideas about mental disorder have broadened during the past two or three decades concomitant with an increase in the possibilities for treatment. People know about tranquilizers and about psychotherapy in its various forms and have to assume, rightly or wrongly, that discomforts like sleeplessness, palpitations, and fatigue are not an inevitable part of the human condition. There is a label that subsumes them—neurosis—and thereby recasts them as symptoms of an illness. If they are now illness, "cure" may be possible.

Something like this happened during and after our survey in the Sine-Saloum. The Serer began to reformulate their discomforts within a medical framework; I suspect they will soon invent new labels to add to their lexicon of illnesses.

Another process was at work, swelling the tissue of village life with the edema of illness. Bodily illness became, in a sense, a metaphor for other life problems. Our medical teams observed that, village by village, the numbers of people who came asking for help varied tremendously. The teams were also struck by differences in the style of asking for medical attention. In the villages we had previously judged to be more socioculturally intact, complaints and demands for service were minimal. People who did come for attention tended to be succinct in describing their problems and, once examined, to take their medicine and leave. In the villages that were changing, people complained more about their health, and, when they came for help, they tended to linger and to engage the medical teams in discussions about their problems in general. In a sense, what we were seeing was a "village hypochondriasis." People were not making up symptoms; what they were doing was learning that symptom language was one language we seemed able to understand. Whatever the source of their distress—poor soil conditions, unjust taxes, or a concern that too many young people were leaving the villages—if they could translate this into disease language, there was a chance we would listen and understand.

DISCUSSION

McDermott and his colleagues (9), working in a cross-cultural situation on the Navajo reservation, raise an interesting question about an experience like ours. They ask: Do "the particular observations that have to do with working with a people represent research findings that have generality, or [do] they merely represent experience, and a certain wisdom presumably acquired thereby, but [which] must remain an essentially individual affair"? In the 15 years since McDermott's article appeared, others have written about how social and cultural factors, when unheeded, spell failure for medical and public health programs in developing areas (10). General themes emerge from this literature, and I believe that these generalizations are finding their way into the curricula of schools of public health and medicine. The bulk of this work addresses itself to service programs; the question of the impact of research projects in developing areas has been relatively neglected. I do believe, however, that general principles relating to research can and must be articulated.

Sampling is one such issue. An accepted technique in the social sciences, and a perfectly feasible method in many settings, drawing a sample from a total population created difficulties for the Serer and presumably could do so in other interdependent, close-knit communities. Were we to do such a study again, my colleagues and I agree we would sample villages as we did before, but we would have to be prepared to examine everyone in the village, in order to avoid singling people out. The expense, of course, would increase, but this is a fact of life and culture, which funding bodies should recognize.

Another issue, a more serious one, concerns the relationships among members of the research team itself. Although the research was carried out under the auspices of the Ministry of Health for Senegal, the research team, while it included a Senegalese anthropologist and a Senegalese psychiatrist, was top heavy with Europeans and North Americans. Africans filled the roles of interpreters and assistants. Thiere, a member of the Serer Royal Family, was one of the most important of our assistants. He introduced us in the villages, acted as an interpreter, and smoothed over many rough spots for us. In matters of proper social conduct, Thiere was perfectly willing to guide and instruct us—but not to tell us where we were going wrong. Part of this is because Thiere's Serer upbringing taught him not to openly criticize others. Because of this, he found it easier to try to excuse our behavior to the villagers than to tell us that our medical teams were offending people. Part of Thiere's reticence stems from the relationship, an inevitably ambivalent one, which is established between Euro-American research workers and the people who work as our guides and interpreters.

The Serer slang term for my European colleagues and myself—"Patron" (Boss)—sums it up. For if "patron" implies a relationship of authority, it also has its pejorative side. The "patron" acts as he does because he knows no better and, lacking the proper education, he can probably never learn how to behave correctly. To Thiere and his friends, we often appeared to be what Alexander Leighton (personal communication) has called "simple fools."

The last concern, and the most serious, stems from the earlier question I raised about the responsibility of a research team to the subjects of the research. Approaching the question from a slightly different perspective, we might ask, "For whose benefit should research be done?"

In *Custer Died for Your Sins*, Vine Deloria (11) berates social scientists for carrying out research that bears no relation to potential service. His remarks, shot through with an incisive irony, provide a warning for all research workers, social scientist and health professional alike: "Anthropologist comes out to Indian reservations to make observations. During the winter these observations will become books by which future anthropologists will be trained so that they can come out to reservations years from now and verify the observations they have studied" (p. 24).

Our own study addressed itself to planning needs at the governmental level. At another level of responsibility, however—the village—the best we could do was to avoid making any verbal promises we felt we could not honor. We stressed the idea that the study would not produce any immediate benefits but that results would be useful for long-range planning. This did not satisfy the villagers.

The need to integrate research and service has been reiterated so often that it has become a cliché. This is unfortunate because clichés convey no sense of urgency. Yet the issue is a very urgent one.

I take some satisfaction in knowing that the results of our research have contributed to the health planning at the governmental level in Senegal. To the Serer villagers, however, this must seem a remote satisfaction indeed. The result of their participation, to many of the Serer, has been disillusionment.

Hans Guggenheim, of the Wundermann Foundation, offers some cogent thoughts relating to the responsibility to people at the village level:

1. The purpose of an inquiry must be made clear as possible to a population.

2. If the community will profit directly from the purpose of the inquiry it can contribute its time. Example: Should a dispensary be constructed?

3. If the purpose of the inquiry is too abstract to be grasped by the villagers, and if no concrete, tangible benefits will be derived by the population within a specified time, then all indi-

viduals who participate in the research should be paid.

4. In integrated communities which continue to have a sense of identity, payment could be made not to the individual, but to the group. For example, a contribution to the local school or hospital, the gift of a well, etc.

Obviously, this does not solve all the ethical problems raised by research nor does it do much to help solve the financial constraints within which one has to work. Indeed it makes research more expensive both in time and in money. Perhaps we should invent a new expense account category such as "population rights compensation" [personal communication].

It is, of course, possible to handle the situation in quite a different fashion. I can well imagine someone taking a position something like the following: "This research was carried out for the benefit of the Serer people as well as for other people in Senegal. The problem is that the Serer are not able to conceptualize this; in their need to see something which has immediate, tangible benefit, they cannot deal with more distant goals." One could then produce a more or less "official" formulation from the social science literature such as: "Primitive people lack future orientation." Explaining away the behavior of others in this fashion acts as a powerful bromide, but is, in the long run, counterproductive.

If research is done for the benefit of a people, the benefit must make sense within their frame of reference. When the Serer perform a fertility ritual or healing ceremony, they do so in the expectation of immediate benefit. Our research rituals—administering questionnaires, doing physical examinations, drawing blood samples, etc.—probably arouse the same kinds of expectations. If, in fact, we cannot fulfill such expectations, in the manner suggested by Guggenheim, we cannot expect people like the Serer to continue to cooperate with us—and we probably should not ask them to.

REFERENCES

1. Reverdy, J-C. *Une Société Rurale au Senegal.* Aix-en-Provence; Centre Africain des Sciences Humaines Appliqúees, 1969.
2. Beiser, M., Benfari, R.C.B., Collomb, H., and Ravel, J.L. Measuring psychoneurotic behavior in cross-cultural surveys. *J. Nerv. Ment. Dis.,* 163: 10–23, 1976.
3. Office de la Recherche Scientifique dans les Territoires d'Outre Mer. *Déroulement de l'Enquete et Resultats Socio-Demographiques de l'En-*

quete Collaborative sur la Sante Physique et Mentale des Serer, B.P. 138. Dakar, Senegal: O.R.S.T.O.M., 1970.

4. Beiser, M., Ravel, J.L., Collomb, H., and Egelhoff, C. Assessing psychiatric disorders among the Serer of Senegal. *J. Nerv. Ment. Dis.*, 154: 141–151, 1972.

5. Beiser, M., Collomb, H., Ravel, J.L., and Nafziger, C.J. Systemic blood pressure studies among the Serer of Senegal. *J. Chronic Dis.*, 29: 371–380, 1976.

6. *Nuremberg Code: U.S. v. Brandt et. al., Nuremberg Military Trials, Oct. 1946-April 1949.* Reprinted in I. Ladimer and R. Newman, *Clinical Investigations in Medicine: Legal, Ethical and Moral Aspects.* Boston: Law Medicine Research Institute, 1963, pp. 116–119.

7. United States Department of Health, Education and Welfare. *The Institutional Guide to DHEW Policy on Protection of Human Subjects.* Washington, D.C.: Dept. Health Education and Welfare, Publ. No. (NIH) 72–102, Dec. 7, 1972.

8. Beiser, M. Definitions of mental illness in tribal Africa and rural North America. Presented at annual meeting of American Anthropological Association, New York, November 19, 1971.

9. McDermott, W., Deuschle, K., Adair, J., Fulmer, H. and Loughlin, B. Introducing modern medicine in a Navajo community. *Science*, 131: 197–205, 280–287, 1960.

10. Paul, B.D. *Health, Culture and Community.* New York: Russel Sage Foundation, 1955.

11. Deloria, V., Jr. *Custer Died for Your Sins.* New York: Avon, 1970.

The Patient, His Culture, and His Art

OTTO BILLIG

The content and symptoms of psychopathological behavior may differ in various cultures. While some conditions are culture-bound and limited to circumscribed areas, as arctic hysteria or amok, other more basic syndromes appear universally in all cultures. Statistical reports of mental illness, however, vary considerably in different countries, as sociocultural attitudes seem to bias the prevalence of diagnostic labels. The diagnosis of manic-depressive psychosis is made 10 times more frequently in Great Britain than in the United States, where schizophrenia is diagnosed far more frequently (1). Such wide variations raise questions as to the reliability of diagnostic labels. It may be of greater significance to determine the primary core features of a psychosis that deal with the patient's ability to differentiate and integrate his concept formations and that illuminate the structure and organization of his thought processes (2). If in discussing such conditions, the term "schizophrenia" is applied, it is important to be aware of the expressed reservations and the wide variations concerning its use.

The schizophrenic personality disintegration disrupts the linkage of thoughts, creating neologisms of temporary significance that interfere with the patient's verbal communication; in cross-cultural studies, local languages may increase the existing difficulties. In culturally isolated areas, the fears and distrust of one's neighbors prevented a linguistic exchange and perpetuated the societal exclusiveness. In some areas of Africa and Asia, a language may be spoken only by small groups of people. In New Guinea, the outsider depends on interpreters (as it is impossible to develop the facility to speak the 700 different local languages) unless the investigations are limited to small areas.[1] But even the best are unable to translate the language of the schizophrenic literally as his words have highly personal meaning, full of overlapping concepts and pathological sentence structures.[2] It becomes almost pathognomic when the interpreter, who may have little difficulty in translating the orderly constructed language of integrated patients, becomes perplexed at his inability to follow the verbiage of the disintegrated personality.

Verbal language requires the ability to arrange concepts in a linear sequence; it dismantles the multidimensional and simultaneous forms as they exist side by side in space and shapes them into a linear order (4). The process is essential for deductive thinking as it leads from one concept to the next as determined by the order of its system (5); it makes it possible to form new, creative links that can be accepted as they interlock with the established total design.

Read (6), Giedion (7), and others believe that visual language existed prior to verbal language as a primary form of communication. It may be assumed that early man during the paleolithic age did not possess the necessary skills to transform the existing multiple, simultaneous concepts into the linear concepts required for verbal language—"art comes into existence as soon as human society comes into existence" (6). Art had forceful meaning for the societal group for which it was created; otherwise, it would have been insignificant. The prehistoric, and particularly the primitive, image-maker was bound by traditional

---

[1]The wide range of traditional patterns, family structure, and art styles in even nearby villages made it desirable to collect material from the various districts of New Guinea rather than to restrict our study to small regions.

[2]The clinician often has considerable difficulties in understanding a schizophrenic's expressions in his own language (3).

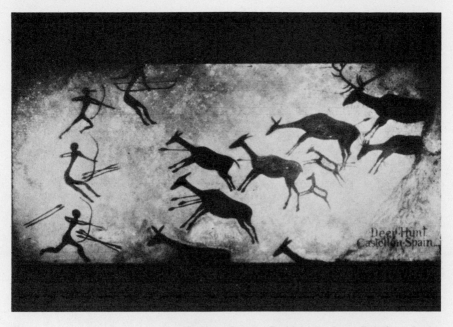

1   Hunting Scene, Prehistoric Cave Painting, Spain

conventions that were rigidly applied and not to be altered (8); colors and forms had specified values.

The works were often hidden in caves, painted on rocks (7); being placed beyond a readily accessible viewing area made a decorative function unlikely. Prehistoric and primitive art served spiritual, mostly magic purposes. It showed hunting scenes (Figure 1) and the animals that were man's prey; at later periods, fertility figures appeared (Figure 2). The art of prehistoric and of primitive man touched on the intrinsic elements of human nature; his masks, his ancestral figures were sacred images that invoked the visual presence of their ancestral spirits. By appearing in the carvings or in the paintings, such sacred images bridged the gap between man and his ancestral world. Their presence allied the supernatural powers in meeting the dangers of a world that was mainly unknown; they served to protect him in warfare, to be there when the young initiates dedicated their lives to the clan and its ancestors. Early art called on the spirits for support to meet and to

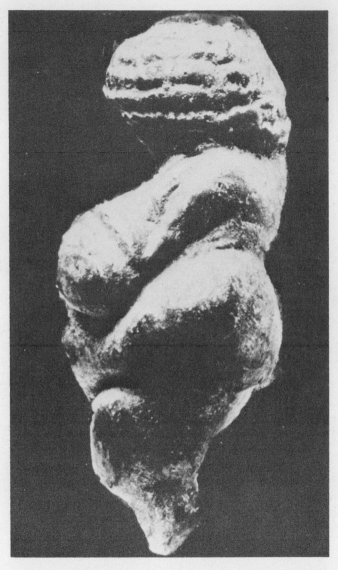

2   Venus of Willendorf, Prehistoric Fertility Figure, Austria

bind[3] the unmanageable anxieties and threats arising within man. To meet his anxieties effectively, man must visualize the helpful hand

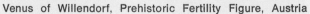

[3]The roots of the word "religion" are found in *ligare* meaning bind and *re* meaning back.

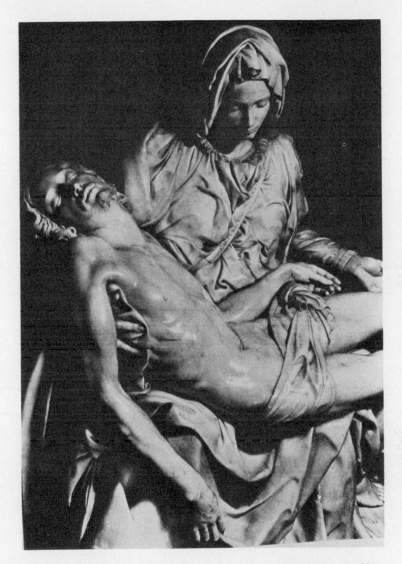

Michelangelo, *Pieta*

3

of the protective powers. As they seem intangible, he produces the
divinities and demons through his art.

The magic force of artistic imagery is found in almost any society.
Western man has a long tradition of being inspired by the sacred
statues and by the paintings of his saints which decorate the altars of
his churches (Figure 3). Repeated efforts to suppress icons as idolatrous

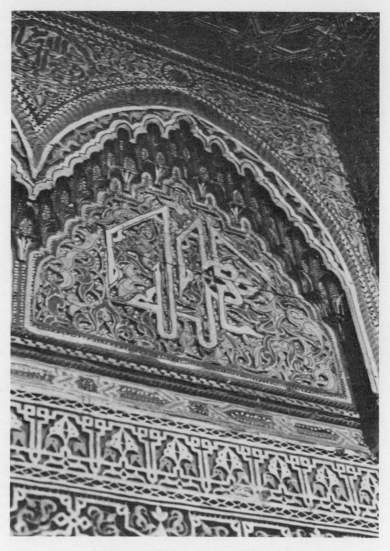

4

Decorative Writing from the Koran, Meknes, Morocco

activity failed (as the Council of Hieria attempted to do in the eighth century). The Koran forbids the making of images as the "abomination of Satan's handiwork," but the mosques are decorated with abstract mosaics and chiseled calligraphy of quotations from the Koran (Figure 4).

Like primitive man, the schizophrenic seeks to express his inner needs and wants by his graphics. One of our patients, a college-educated woman of 22 years, came to the interviews and sat silently during most of the treatment sessions. Visibly frightened, she occasionally expressed her severe apprehensions: "I feel like an ameba . . . jellylike . . . I have no substance . . . I am floating into space." She sat almost motionless as she feared that her inability to control her motions would cause her to float into space where she would dissolve. The "lack of substance" is expressed in shadowlike figures lacking inner details, which she repeats in more than 100 oil paintings; she uses the same patterns in painting shadows standing isolated in an empty space (Figure 5). Her figures are competently drawn and do not lack adequate technical skill as the simple outline and the empty space may suggest. The repetitious sameness of the many paintings indicate the patient's concern to stabilize, at least temporarily, her elusive thoughts through her paintings. She attempts to anchor the fleeting thoughts to the canvas and, not unlike magic art, she makes visible what she fears.

The personality disintegration disrupts the linear sequence of thought processes. A patient becomes unable to shape stable, cohesive thoughts that have a constant position in the hierarchic order of the existing surrounding space (2). Its previously protective boundaries break up; the patient withdraws emotional energy with which he had endowed reality (9), resulting in a pronounced change of spatial relationships. The formerly integrated space loses its depth and plasticity. At first, it appears empty and flat, often limitless and infinite (10, 11). Space and reality appear as a vast wasteland in which the patient feels isolated and alone (Figure 6). As the illness advances, the cohesive order of his world disintegrates further; inappropriate and opposing ideas can no longer be repressed while concurrent and supportive elements are not reinforced. Disproportionate, poorly structured, inarticulated concepts reach conscious levels while integrated, cohesive entities are lacking (Figure 7). The ability to merge images into cohesive patterns becomes lost; concepts are loosened and in a state of flux (4). The fluctuating thoughts are of transient significance and are dependent on the immediate level of personality integration. If the personality becomes better integrated, the earlier delusions become detached and lose their meaning. One of our patients could only vaguely recollect her earlier delusions and, simultaneously, she could no longer attach any significance to her earlier thoughts (Figure 8). As a patient becomes painfully aware of his inability to express the crowding of his multiple thoughts, he begins to draw and paint to overcome his isolation.

Previous publications have attempted to demonstrate that the level of personality disintegration parallels the disintegration of space in the graphics by schizophrenic patients (12). Drawings made by patients at different levels of psychotic disintegration seem to correspond to the

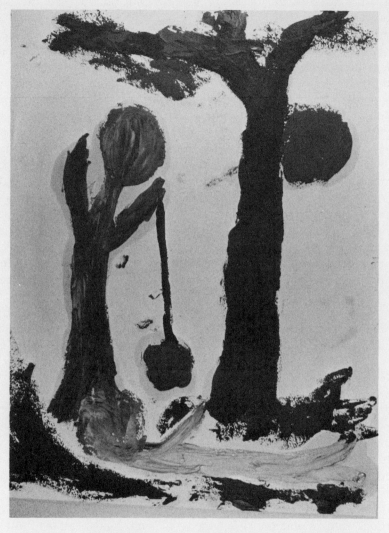

5   Shadowlike Figures, Withdrawn Female Schizophrenic, U.S.A.

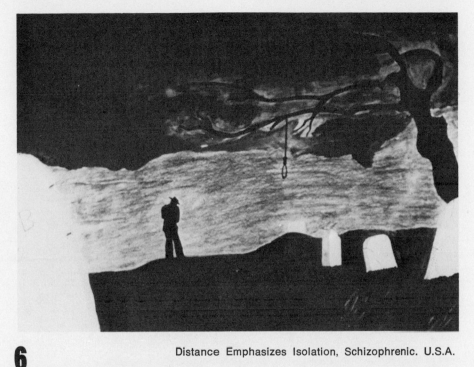

6

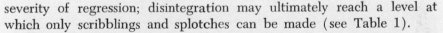

Distance Emphasizes Isolation, Schizophrenic. U.S.A.

severity of regression; disintegration may ultimately reach a level at which only scribblings and splotches can be made (see Table 1).

In order to evaluate the degree of psychotic disintegration, one must be aware of the obvious conclusion that the psychosis develops within a specific cultural setting; the nonpsychotic traditional art must be considered as the cultural root from which a patient's graphics originate. The art style of a specific region appears as a form of expression related to the existing cultural and social influences (13). As long as patients are not severely disintegrated (Figure 9), the content and structure of their graphics are greatly influenced by elements of their own culture. In cases where considerable enculturation has occurred, graphics are produced in Western style (Figure 10).

Subtle structural changes may be overlooked at first and hidden by cultural elements (Figure 9). As regression progresses, pathological structural characteristics emerge more clearly; cultural influences recede and universal culture-free patterns appear. Disintegration leads to a "return to an archaic psychic organization" (2). We have demonstrated

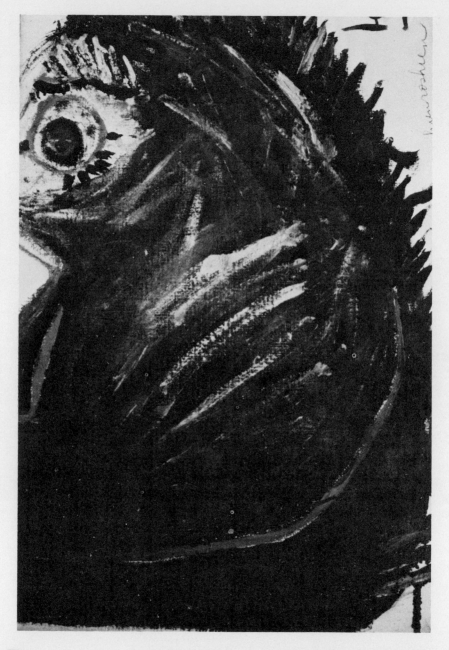

7   Inarticulated Concepts, Regressed Male Schizophrenic, U.S.A.

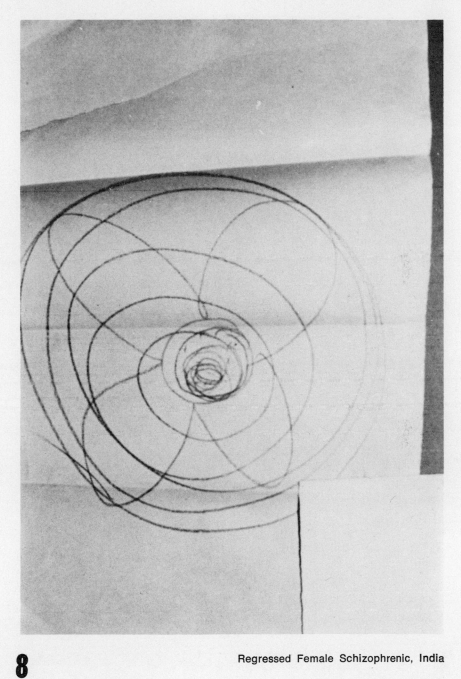

8

Regressed Female Schizophrenic, India

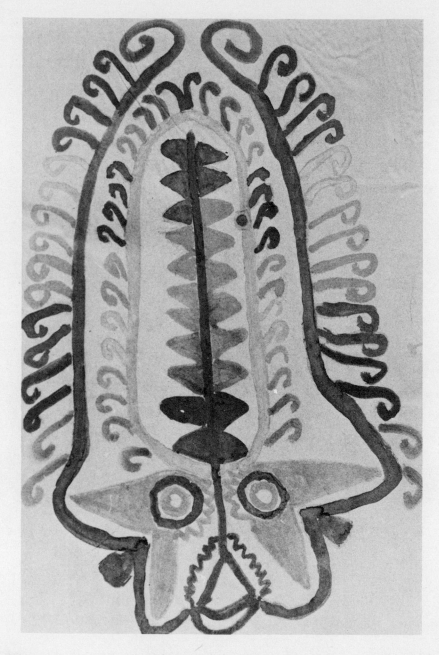

Slightly Distorted Design, Gulf District, New Guinea

Table 1
Regressive Levels of Disintegration

Clinical Condition	Spatial Structure
Beginning withdrawal of object cathexis	Emptying space; shadowy figures; elongation and distortions
Disintegration of ego boundaries	Perseveration; spatial relations destroyed
Inadequate balance between outer and inner reality	Impoverished and condensed design; mixing of planes; "X-ray" pictures (transparencies); vertical projection
More advanced disintegration of ego boundaries	"Horror vacuui"; fragmentation of concepts
Appearance of global concepts	Inarticulated structures
Severe repression of reality relations	Baseline with vertical direction; geometric designs; abstract mandalalike designs
Oceanic feelings	Multidirectional space; "scribblings"

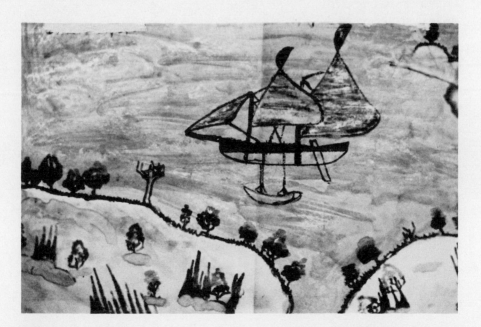

10 Westernized Schizophrenic, Not Severely Regressed, New Guinea

11

Severely Disintegrated Male, New Guinea

in previous reports the regressive patterns of culture-bound concepts (3). New Guinean designs disintegrated to abstractions or to near scribblings (Figure 11) that can be found in graphics by schizophrenics of any culture, Nepalese (Figure 12), African (Figure 13) and Americans alike (Figure 14).

Most of New Guinea and the rural areas of some African nations have remained isolated until recently. We must appreciate the sudden impact of Western civilization on these people to understand its extensive effect on their lives. Many middle-aged New Guineans spent their formative years in complete isolation without ever seeing an outsider. The rough terrain and linguistic differences supported the cultural isolation; the people of the Highlands did not know that other individuals existed beyond a 25-mile radius (14). In many districts, art played a highly significant role in their traditional life, far more than in most

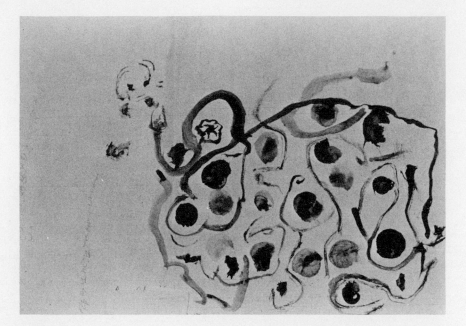

12

Severely Disintegrated Male, Nepal

other cultures. The traditional influences on an individual patient persisted as long as the personality structure was not severely disintegrated.
A patient from a small village in the Papuan Gulf,[4] isolated from
outside contacts, maintained the characteristic features of the traditional
Hohao plaques of his region (Figure 15) during the early stages of
his illness (Figure 16). As his illness progressed, his watercolors showed
decreasing cultural influences (Figure 17), but were somewhat similar
in basic design to the graphics of a Western patient (Figure 18). The
advanced regression caused universal patterns to emerge (3), which
corresponded to the appearance of universal clinical symptoms (16, 17).
The graphics of another patient from the Highlands changed from highly
disintegrated, widely used mandalas and spirals (Figure 11) to pictures of
lizards and crocodiles, a frequent subject in New Guinea art (Figure 19).

---

[4]Detailed clinical findings cannot be discussed here due to lack of space, but
they appear in another publication (15).

13   Severely Disintegrated Male, Kenya

Some areas of New Guinea had been under European control for several generations; the elders of today's patients experienced a state of confusing transition as many of their traditional beliefs came under attack. Their ceremonials, a more obvious expression of their faith, were open to direct attack by zealous missionaries; as a result, the ceremonials disintegrated readily while their faith in the spiritual world continued. Being deprived of the relief obtained by their customary rituals, they felt puzzled. The technological skills of their "masters" added doubts about their traditions and furthered the disintegration of their societal structure. Often humiliated (18), they could not support their children in maintaining the values on which their society was built. The societal disintegration led to the abandonment of serious tribal art work; what remained was mainly "airport art" (19). Such attitudes caused patients who had experienced prolonged European contacts to include Western rather than culture-bound elements in their graphics, regardless of the level of their personality disintegration (Figure 10).

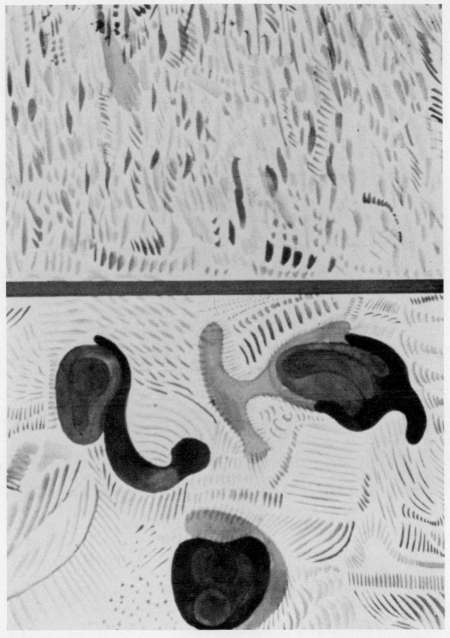

14   Severely Disintegrated Male, U.S.A.

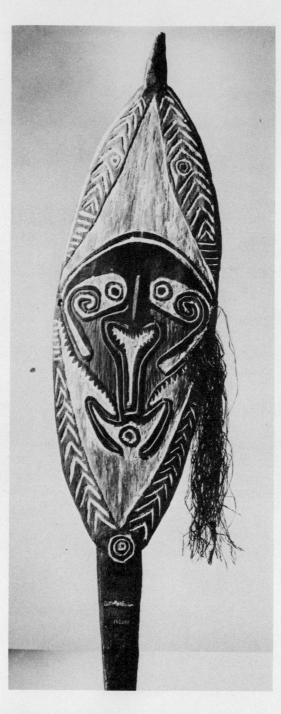

15 Traditional Hohao Plaque, Gulf District, New Guinea (by permission of the Field Museum of Natural History, Chicago, Illinois)

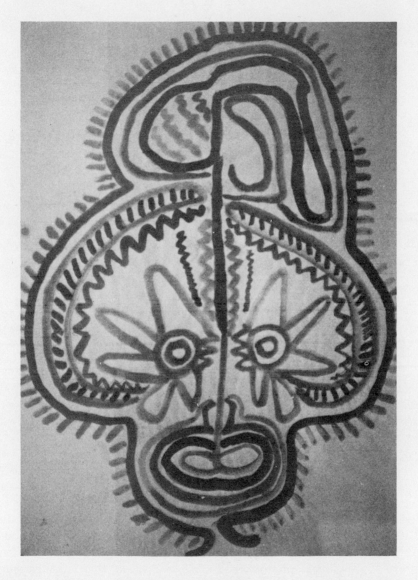

16   Moderately Disintegrated Male Schizophrenic, Gulf District, New Guinea

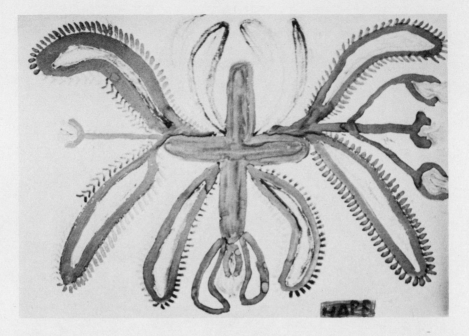

17   Severely Disintegrated Patient (same as in Figure 16)

For comparative studies, we added graphics by patients from entirely different cultural backgrounds. Some were produced by patients from Kenya who came from widely scattered rural areas.[5] Most of them had never had any experience with art and had never used any form of art material. In contrast to New Guinea, art plays a negligible role in the cultural life of the people. Masks are rarely used by any of their tribes and they possess almost no ancestral carvings, in contrast to West Africa where art is of major importance. At most, some of the East African tribes decorate themselves with bracelets and necklaces of no artistic value (20). Yet, disintegrated patients find it easy to draw and paint; some do not need any instructions and encouragement. Highly regressed individuals produce scribbles similar to those by patients from other countries (Figure 13). One patient, diagnosed as schizophrenic, was regressed, semi-mute, and his speech was incoherent; but

[5]By courtesy of Dr. Edward L. Margetts now of Vancouver, Canada, formerly of Nairobi, Kenya.

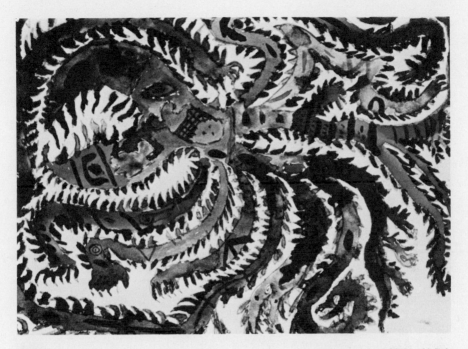

18

Disintegrated Male, U.S.A.

he had no difficulty using crayons which he had not used before. He drew a "calabash" (Figure 20); the brown center represents a chicken; the round circles on the periphery are eggs. The chicken in the drawing can be seen through the transparent rind of the calabash. Patients of Western (Figure 21) and non-Western (Figure 22) cultures paint similar transparent objects or "X-ray" pictures (see Table 1).

We collected additional paintings from a very different area—Nepal. Nepal has a long history of art, reaching back to the third century B.C.; its richest periods were between the fifteenth and eighteenth centuries. While the shrines and temples are filled with spectacular carvings, its art did not play the intimate role that New Guinean art had in the lives of its people. In the Melanesian islands, every adult male had continued contacts with masks and plaques; the men lived with them in the Haus Tamberan[6] where they were surrounded by masks and

[6]Prior to the European penetration, adult men lived in the ceremonial houses discussing the affairs of the village, planning war raids, ceremonials, etc. Masks and sacred carvings were kept in the dark recesses of the meeting places.

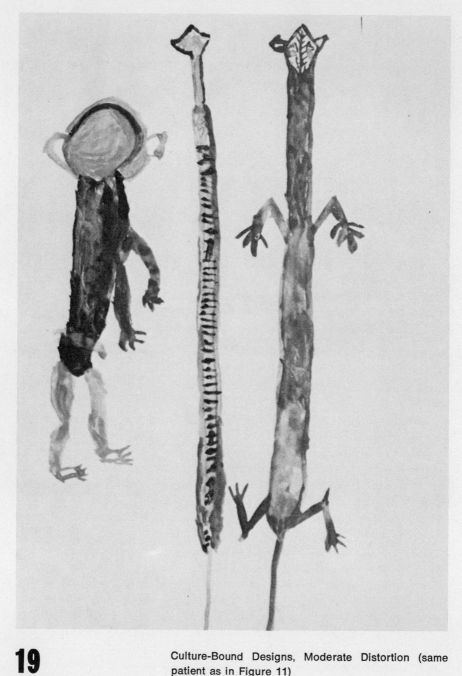

19   Culture-Bound Designs, Moderate Distortion (same patient as in Figure 11)

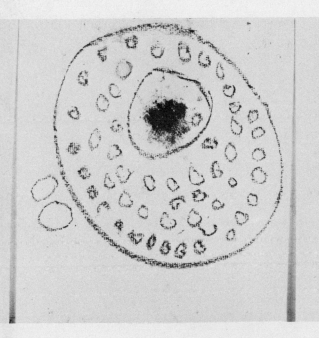

20   Calabash with Chicken in Center, Regressed
Schizophrenic, Kenya

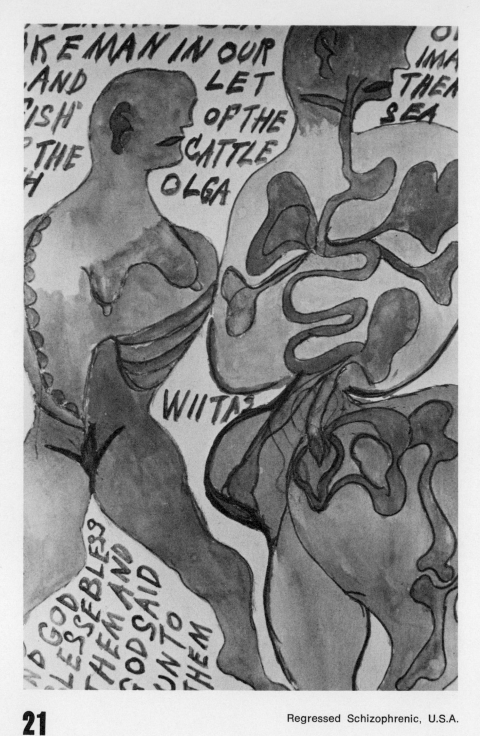

21

Regressed Schizophrenic, U.S.A.

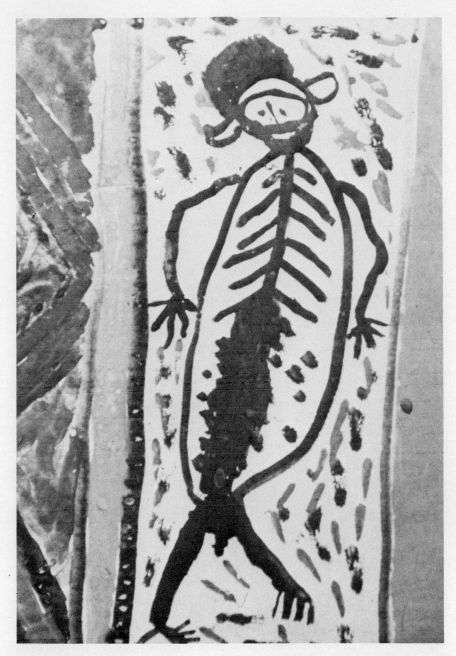

22

Disintegrated Male, New Guinea

plaques. In Nepal, as with religious art in Western cultures, most art is kept in the temples where the worshipper is exposed to the imposing statues of his deities (Figure 23). Nepalese patients incorporate religious ideas in their delusions and hallucinations; some believe themselves to be Lord Shiva, others identify with the other gods. In spite of the obvious presence of religious art and architecture, religious or spiritual content is not prevalent in patients' paintings. New Guineans, on the other hand, seemed to have absorbed artistic concepts as they lived surrounded by their masks and plaques; often the entire community took part in making them (21). Having been exposed to art continuously, patients assimilated the artistic concepts and included them in their paintings when they became mentally ill. In Nepal, art is the work of a professional and meant to be seen principally in the temples and shrines. For the average population, the deities are to be worshipped, but they do not paint or carve them.

The Nepalese graphics were obtained from patients who were hospitalized in the psychiatric division of the General Hospital at Kathmandu.[7] One watercolor has simple forms using pale colors outlining a diamond and, apparently, a flower bed below it; writing, as in the graphics by disintegrated patients from most countries, appears on the right (Figure 24).

Another graphic by a regressed schizophrenic shows circles or splotches mostly of reddish-brown color; they are surrounded by inter-connecting lines, being basically an amorphous figure; some unidentifiable scribblings appear on the left (Figure 12).

A better-integrated patient paints a landscape of high mountains designated by the patient as sunrise in his village (Figure 25). The Himalayan Mountains dominate the scenery in most parts of Nepal and the patient's watercolor must be considered to be culture-bound. The country's high mountains inspire awe in the people; they are seen as unapproachable, mysterious giants to be considered as gods. The highest of them, Mount Everest, Sagarmatha in Nepalese, is translated as "Mother Goddess of the Land"; Annapurna is named the "dispenser of food" since it supplies dependable streams of mountain water when the rivers of the lower lands dry up (22).

The next watercolor (Figure 26) resembles American folk art paintings even though it lacks adequate cohesion. The individual parts of the painting are not integrated into the total concept; they are separated. The painted objects are elevated, distorting the perspective view (see Table 1) and appearing in vertical projection (12) and in a two-

---

[7]We are very grateful to Dr. Sharma, the Chief Psychiatrist at the Kathmandu Hospital.

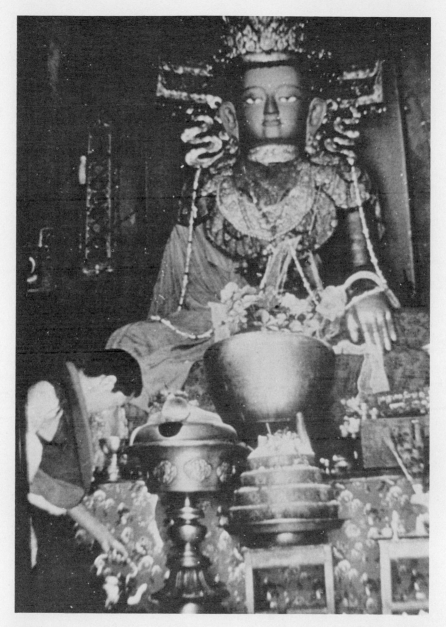

23

Nepalese Shrine

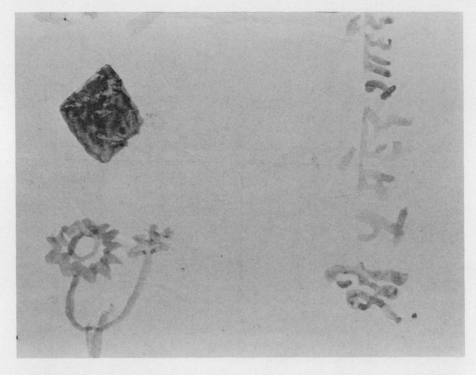

24

Very Regressed Patient, Nepal

dimensional frontal view. Often, folk artists paint landscapes in similar perspective, but their paintings are cohesive and the objects of proportionate size. This patient paints flowers of disproportionate size and a house that is transparent. The rooms seen in the cross-section form isolated squares, and the pathways leading from one room to another suggest some personal meaning to the painter.

A 20-year-old patient who had grown up in Kathmandu, the Nepalese capital, had been hospitalized for two and one half months. He was seclusive and almost unresponsive; he refused to eat and neglected his appearance; his affect appeared flat and he smiled inappropriately. Two figures that appear in his watercolor (Figure 27) maintain a like posture; each carries a sticklike object, pointing in the same direction, and one of the figures is substantially smaller than the other. A duck or bird stands on a rug that is seen top view; other objects, such as flowers and a vaselike container, are seen in side view. The individual

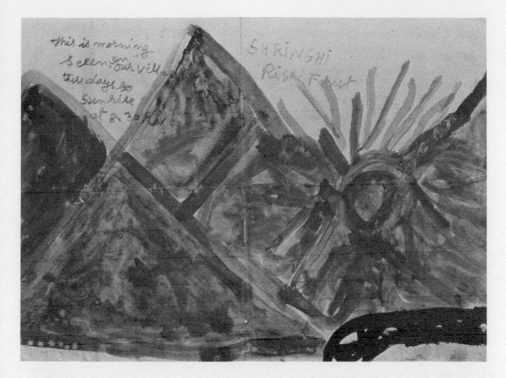

25   Sunrise over the Himalayas, Moderately Regressed
Schizophrenic, Nepal

objects are isolated and not connected with one another. The stippled
bird and rug, as well as the clothes worn by the two men, lend an
oriental impression; other cultural characteristics are missing. The lack
of cohesiveness, the separate disproportioned objects without an inte-
grating background reflect the disintegrated spatial structure observed
in the graphics by schizophrenics from other cultures (23). The graphics
by the Nepalese patients show similar structuralizations of space to
those from other countries. They seem to occur universally—a significant
factor in experiencing reality reaching beyond the limits imposed by
cultural experiences.

In summarizing, the data collected from various countries appear
to support theories of universal factors of behavior—"every man has
numerous latent functions which lead under certain conditions, com-
pulsory and essentially, to the same course ... [psychotic reintegration

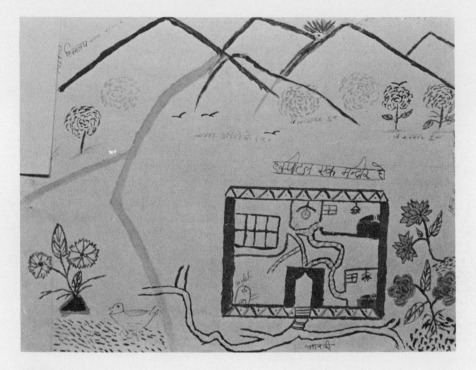

26

Regresed Schizophrenic, Nepal

proceeds] from a state of relative globality and lack of differentiation to a state of increased differentiation, articulation and hierarchic integration" (2). Enculturation exerts a profound influence upon the individual and his society. However, if the personality disintegrates, cultural influences become less significant and more universal elements reappear. As the patient improves clinically, a progressive reintegration can be observed in consecutive drawings, until it reaches the cultural level of the patient's specific societal group. A young American patient who had painted flat, two-dimensional drawings (Figure 28) when she had functioned at a level of marked disintegration reaches a three-dimensional perspective as she reintegrates. The three-dimensional spatial structure has been a characteristic of Western art since the days of the Renaissance art. In contrast, a Melanesian paints plaques (Figure 9) significant of his culture.

It is tempting to conclude that man's concepts of reality are reflected in the spatial structure that he shapes; it tends to develop

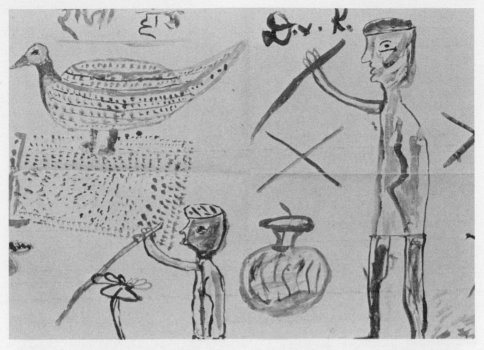

27   Regressed Schizophrenic, Nepal

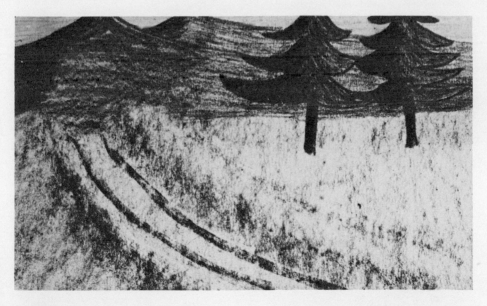

28   Reintegrated Schizophrenic, U.S.A.

universally in various cultures and in very similar directions. Societal demands, socialization processes emphasize and possibly limit the actual levels of reality structure and the view of the world that man can reach within his society.

REFERENCES

1. Zubin, J. A cross-cultural approach to psychopathology and its implications. In: *The Classification of Behavior Disorders,* ed. L.D. Eran. Chicago: Aldine, 1966.
2. Wynne, L.C. The transcultural study of schizophrenics and their families. *Transult. Research,* 15: 10–13, 1963.
3. Billig, O., and Burton-Bradley, B.G. Psychotic "art" in New Guinea. *J. Nerv. Ment. Dis.,* 159: 40–62, 1974.
4. Ehrenzweig, A. *The Hidden Order of Art.* Berkeley and Los Angeles: University of California Press, 1969.
5. Bertalanffy, L. von. *General System Theory.* New York: Braziller, 1968.
6. Read, H. Art in aboriginal society: A comment. In: *The Artist in Tribal Society,* ed. M.W. Smith, New York: Free Press, 1961.
7. Giedion, S. *The Eternal Present: The Beginning of Art.* New York: Random House, 1962.
8. Mead, M. The bark paintings of the Mountain Arapesh of New Guinea. *Technique and Personality,* Lecture Series 3. New York: Museum of Primitive Art, 1963.
9. Federn, P. *Ego Psychology and the Psychoses.* New York: Basic Books, 1952.
10. Burnham, D.L., and Burnham, A.L. *Schizophrenia and the Near-Fear Dilemma.* New York: International Universities Press, 1969.
11. Sechehaye, M. *Autobiography of a Schizophrenic Girl.* New York: Grune & Stratton, 1951.
12. Billig, O. Representation of motion in schizophrenic art. Presented at Fifth World Congress of Psychiatry, Mexico City, 1971.
13. Myers, B.S. *Art and Civilization.* New York: McGraw-Hill, 1967.
14. Forge, A. The People and the Culture. In *Papua, New Guinea.* ed. P. Hastings. Sydney: Angus & Robertston, 1971, pp. 60–73.
15. Billig, O., and Burton-Bradley, B.G. *The Painted Message.* Cambridge, Mass.: A. Schenkman & Halstead Press, 1977.
16. DeVos, G.A. Transcultural diagnosis of mental health. In: *Transultural Psychiatry,* ed. A.V.S. DeReuck. Boston: Little, Brown, 1965.
17. Hallowell, A.I. Hominid evolution, cultural adaptation and mental dysfunctioning. In: *Transcultural Psychiatry,* ed. A.V.S. DeReuck. Boston: Little, Brown, 1965.
18. Ryan, J. *The Hot Land, Focus on New Guinea.* Melbourne: Macmillan Company of Australia, 1971.

18. Beier, U., and Kiki, A.M. *Hohao*. Melbourne: Nelson, 1970.
20. Wassing, R.S. *African Art*. New York: Abrams, 1968.
21. Williams, F.E. *Drama of Orokolo*. London: Oxford University Press, 1969.
22. Hagen, T. *Nepal*. Chicago. Rand McNally, 1971.
23. Billig, O. Is schizophrenic expression art? *J. Nerv. Ment. Dis.*, 153: 149–164, 1971.

13

Cannibalism for Cargo

B. G. BURTON-BRADLEY

The human eating of human beings is by no means confined to exotic peoples, as may be inferred in the conventional descriptions. It is part of the human condition. It occurs as a preferred form of protein consumption or as the result of extreme necessity, to absorb the virtues of others, to facilitate conception, for magicoreligious reasons, in warfare, famine, revenge, filial piety, and justice. Quite unique is the case of cannibalism for cargo reported here in which the eater suffered an overt psychosis before, during, and after the consumption, and whose goal was the acquisition of real and symbolic cargo as exemplified in the Melanesian cargo cult.

The scene of the present account is Tapini in the Goilala country of the Central Province of Papua New Guinea. The people of this area are mountain dwellers who live in small hamlets and grow taro and *kau kau* as their principal diet under a system of shifting horticulture. They are predominantly nonliterate and generally considered fierce

Burton-Bradley, B.G., "Cannibalism for Cargo," JOURNAL OF NERVOUS AND MENTAL DISEASE, Vol. 163, No. 6; 428–431, December 1976, The Williams & Wilkins Co. Reproduced by permission."

and aggressive, a reputation which persists in the minds of many people throughout the country. It is not uncommon in the capital Port Moresby to hear a person say, "I'm afraid of the Goilalas!" The stereotype is, of course, an exaggeration. Many of these fine people now make sterling contributions to the country's development. When one talks to some of the older people, however, they say that in former times one was not considered a man until one had killed someone. And this viewpoint is also held by those convicted murderers whom I have examined and who believe they shine in the eyes of their own people because of their deeds.

CANNIBALISM

With the possible exception of famine, where a single motive is apparent, each act of cannibalism invariably has a multidimensional character. In some instances, a nuclear need arises from famine conditions or other occasional food requirements, but this central feature is usually reinforced or replaced by powerful psychological, social, and cultural factors which are apparently necessary to sustain the custom on a continuous basis.

The word "cannibal" is derived from the West Indies Caribs who were said to be well known for this practice, and since that time "cannibal" has been applied to those developing people from whom the reports came. This is rather a pejorative usage, for the custom is widespread and not unknown in those countries said to have the greatest distaste for it. The prisoners of Belsen ate human flesh (1), as did the survivors of the Andes air crash (2).

In Papua New Guinea cannibalism has been widely practiced in the past, and although by no means unknown in more recent times, the spread of repugnance has tended to reduce its incidence on a regular basis. The Reverend James Chalmers, an early missionary who in 1895 unearthed the legend underlying cannibalism, was himself killed and eaten by the Goaribari people of Papua (3). The men declared they introduced the custom following pressure from the women who were dissatisfied with poor-quality animal protein (4). The Lieutenant-Governor of Papua, J.H.P. Murray, in the early part of the century records how he never could give a convincing reason to the natives as to why they should not eat human flesh (5). And the Government Anthropologist for 20 years, F.E. Williams (6), records how the Orokaiva, a traditional hunter, saw fit to eat perfectly good meat when he could get it without having recourse to the sentimental prejudices of others.

Kuru is a neurological disease occurring in the Eastern Highlands of New Guinea. It is thought to be transmitted by cannibalism (7). It is said to be disappearing now that the people are burying rather than eating their dead.

Payback homicide was an important component of a case of cannibalism coming before the Supreme Court in 1971. This vendetta principle was augmented by the need to shame and insult the opposing clan by eating the victim. The judge ruled that cannibalism was not improper or indecent in the environment in which the accused lived (8). There are many other component motivations for the practice in this country, particularly revenge, but also to absorb the victim's life principle, to facilitate conception, as a part of warfare, and as an act of justice. It is not possible to go into all these motives here, but none of the cases cited in the literature have anything like the distinctive character of the one under review.

CARGO THINKING

Crisis cult activities, wherein a simple technology encounters a more complex one, have been reported from many different parts of the world since Greco-Roman antiquity. The specifically Melanesian form is known as *cargo cult,* a term which appeared for the first time in 1935 as an updated concept and displaced symbol of traditional wealth (9). The central nucleus of all cargo activities is cargo thinking, which may occur in the isolated thoughts of an individual, as in the present case, or, following interaction with others, may find expression in the group actions of many people. It is characterized among other things by a desire for rapid acquisition of material appurtenances by preternatural or other means. It is based on status anxiety and is widespread throughout Papua New Guinea as a specifically Melanesian mode of response. Cargo thinking has tremendous appeal to those in the acculturating situation. It does not occur outside the domain of Melanesian culture, not even in surrounding areas such as Indonesia, Micronesia, Polynesia, or Australia. Other developing countries tend to employ other means. What is characteristically Papua-Niuginian in this subvariety of magicoreligious response to social change is the concept of cargo, the intense individualism, the great concern with wealth both in its overt display and conspicuous consumption, and the multitude of miniature cultural-linguistic groups of which there are some 700.

Cargo thinking serves the emotional needs of the people, and cult development offers a possible alternative, albeit a fantasy one, to the superimposed alien economic system. Historical, religious, economic, and other contextual factors interact with one another and play their part in determining the form a given cult will tend to take but behavior in the long run stems from individuals. There are many variations, and a common type of response is along the following lines. A leader emerges. He announces a great future event, a visual hallucination, or revelation. Preparations are made to deal with the expected changes. New moral and legal codes are put into operation, and that most important of status symbols, new clothing, may be adopted. Airstrips, helicopter pads, wharves, and storehouses are constructed in preparation for the ancestral spirits to bring in the highly prized cargo. Money is destroyed, pigs are killed, and work ceases, for it is felt that these will no longer be needed. When the expectations fail to eventuate, the cult wanes and becomes latent. Those who predicted disappearance of the cults in modern times have often been embarrassed by reappearance of new modifications.

ANAMNESIS

On August 23, 1973, a 30-year-old male Goilala was committed for trial at the district court in the area on a charge of willful murder of his own infant son. When asked for an account of his activities prior to arrest he said, "I want to say some prayers first, and then I will talk to you."

He was educated to the primary third grade at a school where some English was taught, but was insufficiently confident in that language, so examination of his mental state was conducted in the neo-Melanesian pidgin language. He conversed freely. His manner was earnest and cooperative, and he was at pains to try and give an accurate statement of events. His memory showed no major impairment except for part of the period when he had been fasting.

He gave the following account of himself. His father died when he was seven years old. His mother is alive, living in the village. He is the eldest child, and he confirmed his greater load of responsibilities compared with the other siblings. He had three children of his own; two now remain following the sacrifice. He has two cousin sisters (collateral relatives) who suffer from *kavakava* (mental disorder) with histories of aggressive behavior, one of whom was formerly treated at the Laloki Psychiatric Center. He smokes 60 cigarettes per day, and drinks beer, at times heavily to the state of inebriation. He does not "spark" on these occasions, as others do. He is a consistent betel-nut chewer, and averages six to eight chews each day. He is concerned that he did not do so well at school (*"mi no sikul gut"*) and this has been a constant source of worry to him. There are many English words he does not understand, and he carries an English dictionary with him on his person to find out their meaning.

He says he has read many religious books from the Christian Mission and owns a number of these books himself. He has read parts of the Holy Bible, the New Testament, and the Hymn Book in English with the aid of his dictionary. He has also read the catechism in *tok ples* (local language), the prayer book in neo-Melanesian pidgin, and the night prayer book in English and *tok ples*. He remembers particularly one book in English entitled *The New Testament for Modern Man*. He read about John the Baptist and other apostles and about Jesus fasting for 40 days. Following this, he thought a lot about what he could do that would be right for him and his people. He learned about Abraham and the sacrifice of Isaac from the Bible.

After much consideration he resolved on a course of action. He says:

> I decided to kill my child. After I had made up my mind I fasted for five days. I then took my little boy into the bush and came to the place where I had decided to kill him. When I came to the spot, I prepared a small place for the child to sit, and I spread a laplap on the ground for him, then I began to dig a grave. After that was finished, I struck him twice on the forehead with my axe. I then took my knife and cut him in the stomach and upwards towards the chest through the bone. I then took his heart out. I chopped it up and ate some of it. I also made some cuts in my own body and mixed some of my son's blood with this. Then I put the body in the grave. I had brought some glue and petrol with me which I mixed with the remaining cut slices of my son's heart. I tried to boil it but was not successful. I had hoped that the steam and the rest of the mixture would go up to God and he would then send me the power in my dreams to do the right things for my people. The people's heads would also become clear and they would then do the necessary things to bring about the white man's way of life. God would send many goods to the people and we would find money. Then I lay down in the grave and slept with my dead son. No dream came the first night. On the second I dreamed that I saw a light go up to heaven. I then covered the grave and returned to my village.

DISCUSSION

The man whose case is described here is a quiet, reserved person. He has been surrounded on all sides by confusing influences: membership in an aggressive group, introduction of an overseas-style economy, syncretization of Christian religious beliefs, membership in a larger national group with a history of cannibalism and a widespread tradition of cargo thinking, cargo cults, and cargo analogues. He has had to cope with these within the limitations of his own basic equipment. He suffered paternal deprivation at an early period of life. There is a history of hereditary mental disorder in the family. He was trying to emulate component aspects of Christian teachings in order to better his own life and those around him. He misinterpreted the intent of these teachings, but correctly assessed their content and literal meaning.

Given the limited social orbit in which he operated, it might appear that his thinking was normal within this framework. However, the bizarre quality of the act with its morbid mutilating aspects, the family history of mental disorder, the beliefs concerning the sacrifice of his own child which were not held by his own kinsmen, and the inevitable change in body chemistry consequent upon (1) the effect of the acute starvation with its associated ketosis, breakdown in electrolyte homeostasis, and hyperuricaemia, and their influence on the blood supply to the brain (10, 11) and (2) the euphoria of arecolinism in a heavy betel-nut chewer (12), all clearly put the case in the area of abnormality as defined by Western medicine (heteropathology). Knowledgeable informants in the person's own group assure me that the behavior is also clearly abnormal as defined by their standards (autopathology). It seems clear that there was marked autistic thinking and a delusional state prior to the act which were compounded by the starvation and arecoline euphoria at the time of the killing, and that such a combination is consistent with acute schizophrenic reaction. This was followed by remissions and relapses, and when examined 12 months later, the autism and ambitendencies of nuclear schizophrenia were still in evidence.

In Papua New Guinea there are over 50 different Christian Missions all promoting their own separate preferred systems of values; this may create some confusion. Apart from their religious objectives, they have also been active in the health and educational fields, often as pioneers in areas with little government influence. They contain among their members many humane and dedicated people who have devoted their lives to the country, and who have lived under very difficult circumstances. This case raises issues of interest to missionaries generally. Is the current level of communication adequate to provide the information desired? Should scholars translate holy books in their totality, as they do at present, or should they confine themselves to those components that could not be misinterpreted? Or should separate texts be devised that are directed toward the literal meanings of the ethical principles, rather than their symbolic representations? And should they be built from the ground up in conjunction with the newly appearing indigenous scholars? The answers to these questions are of considerable importance to the mental health of the people, and are clearly worthy of close attention.

In a country where the widespread cannibalism of not so long ago has left some small residues at the present time, and where cargo thinking and cargo-cult activities exist, it is not surprising that these two things should come together as they have in the present instance. The man concerned in this case had all the attributes of a cargo-cult leader (13), and all he needed was a deputy, or public-relations man, to transmit his message to the fertile soil of a receptive population, with the possibly serious consequence of a fully developed cult and the social damage this would entail. Fortunately, this did not transpire.

REFERENCES

1. Russel of Liverpool, Lord. *The Scourge of the Swastika.* London: Cassell, 1954.
2. Read, P.P. *Alive: The Story of the Andes Survivors.* Philadelphia: Lippincott, 1974.
3. Ryan, J. *The Hot Land.* New York: St. Martins Press, 1969.
4. Hogg, G. *Cannibalism and Human Sacrifice.* London: Hale, 1958.
5. Murray, J.H.P. *Papua, or British New Guinea.* London: Fisher Unwin, 1912.
6. Williams, F.E. *Orokaiva Society.* London: Oxford University Press, 1930.
7. Glasse, R.M. Cannibalism in the Kuru region of New Guinea. *Trans. N.Y. Acad. Sci.*, 29: 748, 1966.
8. Griffin, J.A. Is a cannibal a criminal? *Melanesian Law J.*, 1: 79, 1971.
9. Mair, L.P. *Australia in New Guinea.* London: Christophers, 1948.
10. Ashley, B.C.E., and Whyte, H.M. Studies in acute undernutrition. *Aust. J. Exp. Biol. Med. Sci.*, 45: 245, 1967.
11. Boulter, P.R., Hoffman, R.S., and Arky, R.A. Pattern of sodium excretion accompanying starvation. *Metabolism*, 22: 675, 1973.
12. Burton-Bradley, B.G. Papua and New Guinea transcultural psychiatry: Some implications of betel chewing. *Med. J. Aust.*, 2: 744, 1966.
13. Burton-Bradley, B.G. *Stone Age Crisis.* Nashville: Vanderbilt University Press, 1975.

14

Folk Therapy in Surinam

EARLINE L. HOUSTON

In June 1974, and again in August 1975, a group of black Americans of the Counter-Evans Expeditions traveled to Surinam to visit the Ndjuka and Saramacca people, two of six black tribes living in the interior. These tribes are the descendants of West Africans brought to the Americas for slavery who successfully fought their captors during 50 years of guerilla warfare. At the request of the colonial government, peace treaties were signed during the 1760's.

Settlements were established along the rivers of the interior preserving many African cultural patterns. Today the tribes number 15,000 to 20,000 people each. The usual village contains some 200 people consisting of a basic group of matrilineal kinsmen, their spouses and offspring. Though the headman and assistant headman of a village owe allegiance to the *Granman* (paramount tribal chief), their social and political influence is limited by a complex set of religious practices, some of which are mediated by *Obiamen* (priest-healers) (1).

We were fortunate to be accompanied by Da Buone, a Ndjuka

Obiaman, to witness some of his work, and to be introduced to others in our travels. The Obiamen do not make a clear distinction between physical and psychiatric illness. Each syndrome described here is explained by a system of retribution for wrongdoing by one of its members for which an entire matrilineage may be responsible. The cure for each illness can therefore be accomplished by re-establishing the balance of merit on the part of the individual or family that has offended the moral order.

Three psychiatric syndromes, their cures, and a funeral (as an example of a generalized cure applied to an entire matrilineage) will be presented. *Fiofio* is a syndrome recognized among the Ndjuka and Saramacca whereby a person may be caused to sicken and even die as a result of negative comments made about him or her. Another syndrome, *Lauw* (perhaps related to the Haitian voodoo *Loa* spirit), is a generalized term for those illnesses in which the individual can be observed to interact with people not present. A third syndrome is called *Didibri Ate* (Devil Heart) in the severe form of which a person wants to do harm to himself or others.

FIOFIO

I was asked to see a 30-year-old woman, pregnant for the sixth time, who complained of vomiting every day for the entire seven months of her pregnancy. She was very thin and neatly dressed in village garb. Physical examination revealed a seven-month pregnancy which was not unusual except that this woman complained of nausea while spitting small quantities of saliva which were blood-streaked on the day of her washing-healing ceremony. During the interview, through an interpreter, the woman kept a sad, pouting expression and a complaining tone of voice. She denied difficulties with her family or in-laws, but admitted that she worried about feeding another child. She spoke with greatest intensity, however, of being insulted by a former friend in her village. This woman had told her that she had the belly of a rat and was getting children she couldn't care for.

Da Buone explained that the pregnant woman had Fiofio caused by the negative statement made by her former friend and invited us to be present at a washing ceremony to safeguard the fetus.

The treatment consisted of literally washing off the effects of the "bad mouth." A circular wooden tray was placed in front of the woman, and a fizzling hot axe was positioned on the ground between her feet. The tray, two feet in diameter, was prepared by marking it with an "X" surrounded by a circle in *pimba dote* (sacred white chalk) as Da Buone prayed to the universe, which is round. An egg was placed in the center of the circle to symbolize the woman's pregnancy. Herbs from the front and back of the house were shredded and added to the tray to symbolize the coming together of the man and woman who made the baby. Finally, calabash spoons, foot-long blades of grass which had been doubled and tied, and three lengths of banana stalk were placed radially around the tray.

The whole was wet and mixed with water and rum as Da Buone prayed and invited everyone to come and get his "bad mouth" off. The villagers came one by one and, using the calabash spoons, grass stalks, and banana shoots, picked up liquid from the herbal mixture. This was sipped and sprayed from their mouths in a fine mist over the woman. Da Buone explained that, just as everything was heated up from the words of the other woman, the hot axe cooled off during the ceremony. He predicted that she might even have a "cool" birth (a delivery without pains). After the spraying, the banana shoots were unrolled and the mangrassi blades were untied while being passed over the woman. Such statements were made as: "Getting children is very important." "The village is getting empty. You are filling the village." "Everyone, the family, the father, the granman, the whole tribe, wants the baby, and that is why it should be born healthy."

The ceremony was interrupted by an argument from another part of the village. People were trying to get the one who had put the "bad mouth" on to come and participate. Da Buone went to join them but returned alone and stated that her coming was not really necessary as the ceremony was effective without her. He sprayed the woman again, squeezed the herbs out over her head, and dropped the egg on the axe, breaking it. Da Buone explained, "As long as the egg is hard, the washing has not gone long enough." He doused the woman with the remainder of the mixture, then with beer. After she left, he sprayed the area with rum, then sprinkled the entire area with white clay. Da Buone later explained that the herbs were used to wash away the "wrong things."

Essentially, the woman was accused by another of wrongdoing for having the arrogance to bring children into the village that she couldn't care for. She agreed with the accusation in that she complained of her poverty and the difficulty of feeding another child, though neither she nor anyone else saw this as the cause of her illness. The washing ceremony was a rebuttal to the accusation and an affirmation of the value of children to the village. It was performed to ensure the health of the woman and child so that they would not suffer from the effect of the "bad mouth."

The syndrome of Fiofio can be seen as analogous to the more

familiar phenomenon of scapegoating. Scapegoating is usually thought to require at least two individuals who reciprocally validate the idea of the "badness" of the third. One of the individuals may be replaced by a critical superego (2). The Ndjuka describe this as a dyadic phenomenon operating only between accuser and accused. They emphasize that the accuser is frequently a former friend, important to the accused, but no definite role is ascribed to a critical superego. Though this was denied, it appears in this instance that the superego of the woman may have been in agreement with her accuser. Surely the cure was a potent group repudiation, both of the critical friend and the critical superego.

LAUW

Da Buone explained, "When someone is sitting and talking to himself, and there is no one with him, [or] he may be hitting things and cursing, you say, 'Ah, he's Lauw.' When you feel bad, so you want to do something wrong or kill someone or something like that, then your bad spirit is working, and then they say that you're Lauw. If you know how to cure him, it's easy to get him back again."

On a visit to the village of Moengo Tapa in July 1974, where several Obiamen were working, I was allowed to witness a fragment of a healing ceremony. A sick woman with a very bizarre expression was sitting on a cloth beside her son. I was told that the woman had a spiritual illness with the same air of significance that I have been told in this country, "She is crazy." The Obiamen split the cloth between them and gave each one a piece as a sign that he had been curing them, and also as a protection to prevent the illness from recurring. The son was part of the ceremony as a sign of the family's consent for the woman to be cured, which was necessary because, according to Da Buone, "If part of the illness gets off her, it must also get off her children."

Pakosi, son of Da Pakosi, a Ndjuka Obiaman, told me that even "if the mother is Lauw and the son is not, the sickness is [regarded as] a family thing. [For example] if the mother died, the son or someone else in the family might get Lauw. A wrong thing [must have been] done by an ancestor. Such things come down through the generations and the children get sick."

"Splitting the cloth" is the same cure as the one used for twins. Pakosi explained, "If we are twins and our spirits are fighting, so that one of us is sick, they'll split the cloth. Or, if we cannot separate and live without each other, they'll split the cloth."

Another cure for Lauw consists of washing. According to Pakosi, "You can kill a chicken, put the chicken in water and wash the person. The Lauw is switched into the chicken that dies. You split the chicken into two pieces. If a certain two organs in the chicken are dark, things are still wrong. If things are okay, the two are white. Also, if they are black, you have a hard job. You have to go back and consult your spirit."

Certain aspects of schizophrenia as it is understood in Western psychiatry are not dissimilar to this description of Lauw and its cures. The nature of the "splitting the cloth" cure for both Lauw and twins that are too close implies a bond between the family members which is integral to the illness. Cure is accomplished by giving the family members symbolic permission to separate.

The notions of pseudomutuality and the double bind in schizophrenia are not inconsistent with this older folk formulation. In both, there are injunctions against divergence from the family pattern, for both the patient-victim and other family members. According to Wynne and his associates (3), pseudomutuality is characterized by:

> a persistent sameness of the role structure of the family . . . an insistence on the desirability and appropriateness of this role structure . . . evidence of intense concern over possible divergence or independence from this role structure. . . . divergence is perceived as leading to disruption of the relation and therefore must be avoided . . . [pp. 207, 209].

Watzlawick (4) notes that the double-bind situation includes:

> a primary negative injunction . . . a secondary injunction conflicting with the first at a more abstract level and like the first enforced by punishments or signals which threaten survival. . . . A tertiary negative injunction *prohibiting the victim from escaping the field* [italics added] . . . [p. 133].

Lauw may also be understood as a scapegoating phenomenon in the tribal culture as (1) Lauw is believed to be retribution for an ancestral wrong for which all the descendants are equally liable, and (2) cure of the victim, whether by "splitting the cloth" or washing with a chicken which is killed and assumes the Lauw, is also believed to remove the threat of Lauw from the rest of the family. There are parallels in Boszormenyi-Nagy's (2) discussion of the assignment of a "bad" role: "Self-paralyzing psychotic behavior may represent aspects of a captive object role assigned by the family system . . . the members of which feel threatened by some implication of evil . . . and who agree to use an Other . . . to impersonate evil" (p. 70).

DIDIBRI ATE

In contrast to Fiofio, caused by someone making bad statements about a person, and Lauw, an illness of the head—a retribution for wrongdoing by an ancestor, Didibri Ate (Devil Heart) takes place within the individual, as Da Buone would say, "deep within the heart."

It is understood to be an unbalancing of the relationships between the self and the two *Yeyes*, the one good and the one bad spirit that walk along with the self. When the good spirit is killed and the bad spirit has won, the person gets Didibri Ate. As such, it is a more serious illness and is much more difficult to cure than Lauw in which the bad spirit is merely in ascendancy over the good spirit.

According to Da Buone, in severe cases of Didibri Ate, wherein someone kills repetitively, cure is difficult or impossible. Often the one who has killed is put into an asylum, but when he is released, he kills again. As Da Buone notes:

It is especially difficult to cure because you don't see the person when he is well. Those people don't mind being like that. Instead of asking to be cured, they try to get courage enough to kill again. Also, those people who feel they are not worth living any longer can't be cured. The Obiaman has to know a lot about the person himself in order to teach him how to be cured or how to serve his two spirits. In Didibri Ate, he has to be taught how to help the good spirit and put down the bad spirit. The person has to know what he has to serve before he can believe it will be possible to change. [Those who are less severely afflicted for instance], those who are sitting and crying, thinking their life is bad and they are no good, or they have no one to look after them because they have no wife or husband, or feel bad because they have done something wrong, can be helped. As long as the Obiaman can talk to them and find out what is depressing them, he can wash them, try to find a companion for them, and talk to them until they see what they have done wrong and promise not to do it again, so they feel better. This is a cure by talking, or *a moffo* (by the mouth).

I presented to Da Buone the case of a family undergoing divorce in which one of the children got ill during the constant bickering of the parents. Seven years before, the father had had another child outside the marriage, but had lied about it, and now was very depressed about the divorce.

Da Buone stated that this was a family affair, not of the man, his wife, and children that we were seeing in treatment, but of the man, his parents, brothers, and sisters. The parents would be instructed to talk with the wife and say, "Listen, it's my son so I am responsible for his faults. I will take care that he will feel sorry and know he has done a wrong thing, and promise not to do it again, if you will take him again." The whole family would then call the man and sit down and curse him. The mother and father would say, "We are responsible, we have made you. We are ashamed you have done such a thing and lied all those years. If you do something like that again and you don't feel sorry, we won't talk anymore with you or take you as our son any longer."

The son returns after several days, says that he sees he has been wrong and is sorry for it. The family talks with the woman and brings them together again. The man tells his wife the same thing. The divorce, the man's depression, and further illness in the child are therefore prevented, according to Da Buone.

There are several assumptions in this description of Didibri Ate: The family is directly responsible for the actions of its members and is a strong, overt force for social control. In contrast to Lauw, caused by the transgression of an ancestor, Didibri Ate is brought about by wrongdoing on the part of the sufferer.

Wrongdoing destroys the balance between one's good and bad spirits. To re-establish that balance or "teach him how to serve his spirits," the task of the healer is to discover the offense, mobilize the resources of the family of origin, so that the sufferer not only repents of his acts in their presence, but also tries to improve. The Obiaman does not cure the illness, but teaches the sufferer how to do this by changing his behavior in order to rebalance his previous wrongdoings.

The relationship between the self and the good and bad spirits that "walk along with" and are kept in balance by the self immediately brings to mind the relationship between the ego, superego, and id and the balance the ego negotiates between one's internalized moral code and one's instinctual impulses. It is of interest that once lost, the balance cannot be regained by merely making a private resolution to be better in the "serving" of one's good spirit. Nor was it ever suggested that one could redefine the moral code (modify a harsh superego). Rather, the emphasis is on actually changing one's behavior toward the wronged others, since that behavior directly destroyed the balance between one's good and bad spirits, thereby causing the illness.

THE FUNERAL

On arrival in Asidon Opo, capital of the Saramacca tribe, we were told that a funeral was in progress. It is not unusual for a funeral to continue for two or three weeks, as this one did, before the body is buried. During this period, several rituals are carried out, some of which are related to the determination of the agents responsible for the death and the symbolic and actual payment of goods to the family of the deceased.

We were told that an avenging spirit (*Kunu*) had just killed the eighth person, a woman, from this family in the last several years. According to the dead woman's son, her brother and two other people killed a man five or six years before, through the use of *Wisi* (*Obia* used for evil). The man went upriver and drowned. The two other people were the man's friend and his wife, who used to boss him around, so that people thought she wanted him dead. The Kunu responsible for the deaths of eight of the woman's family members is the avenging spirit of the dead man, who strikes without discrimination among the family of the ones who killed him unjustly.

For several mornings, children were kept inside their homes while a group of angry young men rushed about the village attempting to tear down the property of those responsible for the woman's death. They were resisted in mock fighting by defenders from the village who would not allow the destruction of the property. Finally, at noon on the last day, the village members went to wash in a bath of herbs to rid themselves of the bad feeling that had been causing the fighting.

In the afternoon the young men who had been out all morning doing the gravedigging returned and carried the casket around the village to the woman's old familiar places. Two other men carried a boat cut in half around to various village members while an elder inquired of the spirit inside, "Was it this one who was responsible for your death, or this one?" According to village belief, the spirit would answer by rocking the boat. Cloth, tobacco, barrels of gasoline, etc., collected from those adjudged responsible for the death, were brought to the central conference house to be given to the family members. Afterward, the woman was buried far from the village. Only men went to bury her, for to avoid the escape of her spirit from the grave, it had to be filled very quickly, and the men had to depart from the area running.

There was nightly dancing and singing to lament the death of the woman. On the last night, the dancing continued until daybreak.

The death of this woman as the result of an act performed by her brother is another illustration of the direct responsibility one matri-lineage member may have for the behavior of another. The brother's responsibility was even greater because he was said to know the cause of her illness (the Kunu), but had said nothing about it, presumably limiting her chances of being saved.

One way of understanding the funeral with its elaborate provisions for detecting the agents of the death and exacting payment from them is to regard the funeral as a generalized cure for suffering before it occurs, because the potential Kunu—the dead woman's spirit—is pacified by the payment to her by those responsible for her death.

DISCUSSION

The consequences of unjust behavior for one's family are far more overt than in Western societies (5). In each of the three syndromes and the funeral described, illness or death is regarded as the result of wrongdoing. Fiofio is caused by wrongdoing by the other who accuses unjustly, Lauw is retribution for wrongdoing by an ancestor, and Didibri Ate is caused by one's own wrongdoing. Cures vary accordingly. The task of the Obiaman is to discover where the imbalance of justice in relationships lies and to make it possible for the victim to re-establish a balance (5). Moreover, the instructions of an Obiaman are in the nature of commands, for unlike Western psychiatrists, the Obiaman also holds the position of priest, human guardian of the moral order.

Wrongdoing by the victim as the cause of illness in the woman with Fiofio seemed less obvious than in the man with Didibri Ate. Though the woman obliquely admitted the truth of the accusation by complaining of the difficulty of feeding another child, the societal emphasis was on the accusation by another as causative of the illness threatening herself and the unborn child. The birth of a healthy child was considered in the best interests of the village. To neutralize the force of the accusation, the Obiaman utilized the power of his position and the symbology of the ceremony to obtain the collective strength of a pardon by the village.

The victim of Lauw is believed to suffer in direct retribution for wrongdoing by an ancestor, retribution for which his other family members are also at risk, and from whom he must obtain consent to be cured. The washing cure rids the victim of the wrong, transferring it into another object which is killed. "Splitting the cloth" is also regarded as curative, with its implicit permission from another family member to separate, to be free of the scapegoat position. The victim of Lauw is cured through the actions of others, the Obiaman and his family, perhaps because he is believed to be suffering for the misdeed of another.

In contrast, in the severely depressed version of Didibri Ate, one's own wrongdoing is seen to cause the death of one's good spirit and to leave one with a feeling of unworthiness to continue living sufficient to cause suicide. In the less severe case described, Da Buone would utilize the family of origin in working out a just solution that acknowledges the responsibility of the individual for changing his behavior and his obligation as a family member.

A great deal of time and concern are given to the complex series of activities that comprise a funeral, for the important task of pacifying a potential Kunu. If one can be sickened or killed by a Kunu for the unjust act of another member of one's matrilineage, one's interest in the justice of the other's behavior is obvious. Reciprocally, one has a huge obligation to behave justly so as not to bring suffering randomly to innocent members of one's matrilineage. Acts of healing, funerals, and the assumptions underlying these rituals serve as powerful reminders of the moral order binding one member of the matrilineage to another.

REFERENCES

1. Price, R. (ed.). *Maroon Societies: Rebel Slave Communities in the Americas.* Garden City, N.Y.: Anchor Press/Doubleday, 1973.
2. Boszormenyi-Nagy, I., and Framo, J. (eds.). *Intensive Family Therapy: Theoretical and Practical Aspects.* New York: Harper and Row, 1965.
3. Wynne, L., Ryckoff, I., Day, J., et al. Pseudomutuality in the family relations of schizophrenics. *Psychiatry,* 21: 207, 209, 1958.
4. Watzlawick, P. A review of the double-bind theory. *Family Process,* 2: 133, 1963b.
5. Boszormenyi-Nagy, I., and Spark, G. *Invisible Loyalties: Reciprocity in Intergenerational Family Therapy.* New York: Harper and Row, 1973.

15

Opium Addiction in Laos: An Overview

JOSEPH WESTERMEYER

This study was supported in part by the Minnesota Medical Foundation, the International Programs Office at the University of Minnesota, and the National Institutes of Drug Abuse (Grant Number 5 TO1 DA00023-02).

The assistance of the following people is acknowledged: Drs. Charles Weldon and Chomchan Soudaly; Messrs. Larry Berger, Vang Tou Fu, and Vang Geu; and Mrs. Gaohli Lyfong.

INTRODUCTION

The Literature

Observers in Laos and adjacent areas of Thailand have stated that opium addiction primarily occurs among the tribal groups who raise the opium poppy (such as the Hmong or Meo), and among the proprietors of urban opium dens (presumably mostly Chinese) (1–3). Two observers (1, 2) have reported that only Meo men were addicted.

Another (3) indicated that "the Lao are rarely addicted to the drug." The implication in these reports is that opium addiction is merely a "cultural" phenomenon without attendant problems in the area of health, family life, economics, or society.

These observations regarding opium addiction in Indochina are quite at variance with reports from China, including Hong Kong. A nineteenth-century author (4) from mainland China recorded that only a minority of Chinese addicts were able to use opium episodically or were able to function reasonably well on regular doses of opium. Both Park (4) and more recent observers (5, 6) have reported that, while opium use may be kept at nonaddictive levels, opium addiction tends to be associated with a wide variety of problems, both for the addicts themselves as well as for their families and society. These include the usual biomedical, psychological, and family problems. More recently legal problems have ensued since opium and heroin became illegal, though even in former times some Chinese opium addicts undertook illegal life styles in order to supply themselves with opium (7).

The Problem

A series of studies was undertaken in order to elucidate these various conflicting reports. Specifically, answers were sought to the following questions: Could opium usage occur without leading to addiction, and if so how prevalent was this phenomenon? Could addictive opium usage be maintained without leading to significant problems for the addicted person, the family, or society? If problems did ensue how frequent and what kind of problems were they? Were there ethnic or sex differences in the incidence of addiction, or in the addictive course? If addiction was problematic, would addicts be interested in seeking treatment? Were traditional forms of treatment available for addiction? How efficacious might modern forms of treatment be for addiction in a society where opium use was traditional?

METHOD

Between 1965 and 1975, a total of three years were spent in Laos during seven separate visits. The first and longest of these visits—undertaken to collect data for a thesis in anthropology—took place during 1965–1967. The research method during that time (8) consisted mainly of anthropological observation and interviewing regarding the raising of opium poppy by Meo farmers, the economics of poppy cash-cropping, and the use of opium by the Meo. A small survey of Meo addicts (9) was taken in order to ascertain the age and sex distribution of addicts. The second project in 1971 consisted of an intensive survey of 40 addicts, with data obtained both from addicts and their relatives regarding demographic characteristics, social and family history, and opium usage (10). Also, a survey of opium dens and "folk treatment" for addiction began on that visit and extended into subsequent visits (11, 12).

During the next four visits from 1971 to 1974, I served as a consultant to the Ministry of Health in Laos as the ministry sought to provide services for the large number of opium addicts who had become refugees as a result of the Indochinese war (13, 14). The establishment of a treatment center for addicts provided an opportunity to obtain demographic and clinical information from a large number of addicts (15, 16). It also provided the opportunity to examine whether treatment for addiction might be accepted by addicts in Laos, as well as to see if treatment for addiction might be efficacious in the Laotian context (17).

A final visit in 1975 enabled me to collect data regarding specific issues that had been raised as a result of earlier studies. In particular, it was of interest to note whether incapacitating psychiatric disorders were associated with opium addiction. Fifty-six addicts from the United States and Europe who had presented themselves for treatment of narcotic addiction at the Laotian treatment facility were also studied (18, 19).

SUMMARY OF MAJOR FINDINGS

Non-addictive Opium Usage

Nonaddictive opium use was observed in Laos. Especially among those who raised opium, the Hmong (Meo), some smoked opium only on festive occasions, such as at New Year's or after traveling some distance to visit friends or relatives. Opium was also used by these same people, as well as by other ethnic groups, as a medication to relieve cough, diarrhea, or musculoskeletal aching. A small survey among Hmong adults (8, 9) indicated that occasional nonaddicted users may outnumber opium addicts, though the numbers were so small as to preclude definitive conclusions.

Several American acquaintances in Laos smoked opium on one or a few occasions without becoming addicted. A few became quite ill from the experience, with symptoms of nausea and vomiting persisting for a few to several hours. Those who took fewer draughts from the opium pipe noted mild symptoms of lethargy, but no remarkable "euphoria." One physician having a bout of diarrhea at the time found that a few pipefuls of opium relieved his condition—much as might a few doses of tincture opium. A few others were unable to inhale the volatilized opium deeply into the lungs and "set" it by a val Salva maueuver (i.e., forcible exhalation against a closed glottus). The latter remarked on the sweet, pungent odor of the opium, but experienced no physiological or psychological effects.

This is not to say that the occasional user does not run the risk of developing opium addiction. Many Hmong, despite the widespread availability of opium and its prevalent usage, refused to ever use opium— even to relieve severe pain, upper respiratory or gastrointestinal symptoms—because of the risk of becoming addicted. Several Hmong informed me that a high proportion of those who use opium do at some subsequent point in their life become addicted; their guesses ranged from "half" to "many" to "most." Surveys of addicts (10, 17) indicated that many persons had used opium for years prior to becoming addicted to it (38 years in the case of one addict). As one old Meo woman put it, "If you never use opium, you never become addicted."

Among my European and American acquaintances, three became addicted to opium as a result of trying it for "a lark" or "just to see what it was like." All three were men who became addicted in their twenties while living and working among indigenous peoples in Southeast Asia. Their case vignettes follow:

A was an American who had been with the Peace Corps in Thailand for two years. He came to work in Laos where he was employed by the International Voluntary Service to work among refugees. While he had found his work in Thailand pleasant and not especially stressful, conditions were much different in Laos. He had to work long hours, seven days a week, assisting refugees in obtaining the basic necessities of life. Moreover, he worked in militarily insecure areas. In the few months following his arrival, two other IVS employees had been killed. Initially he tried opium because of curiosity. After a short time he began to use it regularly and became addicted to it within a few months. Though he hid his opium addiction from other Americans, Hmong (Meo) officials became alarmed at his addiction in view of the major role he played in refugee-relief activities. They informed his American supervisor regarding his addiction, and he was evacuated to the United States for treatment.

B was a lonely individual who had made a tenuous social adjustment prior to leaving the United States, though he had done well academically and possessed a Master's degree in his field. His loneliness and social marginality continued during his teaching at a university in Malaysia. In addition, he had chronic pain and disability as a result of a childhood paralytic disease. Invited by a Chinese co-worker to visit an opium den, he enjoyed the experience, began to repeat it regularly, and thus became addicted. Later he took a job in Laos, where he married a Lao widow, the mother of four children. She gradually became alienated by his increasing opium use, complaining that he spent all of his evenings and weekends in opium intoxication, spent a great deal of the family income on opium, and was providing a poor example for the children. Consequently he sought treatment in Laos for his addiction. At one year post-treatment, he remained abstinent from opium.

C was a European behavioral scientist who had become addicted to opium a decade ago during his first field research among a tribal group that raised opium. Initially he had been mainly curious about observing opium usage. However, after long months of isolation from other Europeans and from urban centers, his host invited him to join him in opium smoking. He liked the experience, soon undertook regular opium smoking, and became rapidly addicted. He remained addicted throughout the remainder of his research activities. As he was leaving the country, he withdrew "cold turkey" from opium smoking, with severe aching and gastrointestinal symptoms that lasted a few weeks, and symptoms of myalgia, dysphoria, and insomnia that persisted several more weeks. During an interim of some years in Europe, he did not seek out narcotics or experience trouble with other drugs. When he subsequently returned to Southeast Asia to again undertake field research, he became readdicted within days of arrival and remained addicted throughout his stay. Again he withdrew himself upon leaving the country to return home. When I met him a few years later at an international conference, he was not abusing any drugs nor did he "crave" opium. Nonetheless, he stated quite affirmatively that he was sure that he would become readdicted upon return to Southeast Asia to resume field work.

In sum, occasional nonaddictive use of opium is certainly possible. It occurs where usage is infrequent and persists only over an evening or a few days' time for ritual purposes or for an acute, self-limited medical problem. However, frequent usage occurring over some weeks places the individual at high risk to more frequent usage and to higher doses—that is, to the development of tolerance and addiction. Though there have been no long-term prospective studies to establish the point, conventional wisdom in Laos suggests that persistent nonaddictive usage —whether for "relaxation" or to "treat" persistent pain, loneliness, dysphoria, or diarrhea—places people at high risk for the development of addiction.

Problems Associated with Opium Addiction

Unlike alcoholism, chronic opium addiction can persist over years and even decades without causing incapacitating or lethal medical problems. This is not to say that addiction does not cause any medical problems, since it is commonly associated with a wide variety of medical problems. First among these is the withdrawal syndrome associated with cessation of opium usage in the addicted individual. Some morbidity occurs in association with withdrawal among all addicts, though symptoms tend to be fairly mild and short-lived among the few who have relatively small addictions. Among those with larger addictions, the morbidity is so aversive to most addicts that they do not undertake "cold turkey" withdrawal on their own. A study done by the Ministry of Welfare in Laos of addicts who received "cold turkey" treatment at a Buddhist wat in Thailand indicated that the mortality of addicts on the way to the wat, while there for a few days, and on the way home was close to five percent (nine deaths at the Buddhist temple and 35 deaths during the trip to the temple and back, among a total of 825 addicts). Even with close medical supervivision at the National Detoxification Center in Vientiane, Laos, there were four deaths among 800 patients over a 15-month period, and a fifth patient died while in withdrawal a few moments after arrival (17). Elderly addicts are at greatest risk of a lethal outcome during withdrawal.

In addition to the morbidity and mortality associated with withdrawal, other chronic health problems attend opium addiction. The most widespread of these is protein and vitamin malnutrition, due to the addict's abandoning eating and the buying of food for the smoking and purchase of opium. Among older addicts who have been smoking for some years, pulmonary problems are commonplace including chronic bronchitis, emphysema, and an acute asthmaticlike condition that sometimes accompanies withdrawal.

Economic problems are also frequent. As the addict increases the time spent in smoking and in intoxication after smoking, less time is spent in economically productive activities. At the same time, as the extent of addiction increases, the addicted poppy farmer consumes more of his cash crop and thus sells less of it in order to purchase other articles. Salaried individuals spend increasingly greater amounts of money on opium. Self-employed individuals (such as merchants or artisans) devote less and less of their energies to their work. Eventually many addicts support only themselves and their addiction, leaving spouse, children, and other dependents to provide for themselves.

Family and marital difficulties are closely related to these economic problems. As addicted individuals spend more money for opium or consume more of their opium cash crop, fewer economic resources are available for the spouse, children, and other family members. Thus, the spouse and children usually have to undertake more economic activities in order to support or care for themselves. The clothes worn by those with an addicted parent or spouse are more apt to be shoddy. Their food is often less nutritious, and an addict's children are less apt to be attending school. Family members complain that their addicted member provides them with less companionship and spends most of his or her time intoxicated on opium. Since opium addiction tends to run in families (10), other family members report that the addicted member serves as a poor example for the children and young people in the family.

Prior to 1970, criminality rarely occurred in association with addiction in Laos (except for burglary by young urban males). However, a serious social crisis developed in the early 1970's as increasing numbers of opium poppy farmers were pushed by war out of their traditional opium-growing areas. At that time Laos probably became an opium-importing country in contrast to its traditional role as an opium-exporting country. Two problems ensued: (1) addicted farmers who had previously raised their own opium now had to purchase their opium; and (2) since Laos was no longer exporting large amounts of opium, and indeed was importing some, the price of opium went up. All of this was further complicated by the fact that in 1971 the government of Laos passed a law forbidding the transport and sale of opium and the registration of opium dens. As a result, opium became even more expensive; and heroin was introduced because it could be more readily smuggled and used surreptitiously (15). All of these factors led to an outbreak of theft among addicts within refugee camps. Considerable strife began to occur within extended families as older addicted patriarchs insisted on reducing the extended family to poverty by buying opium rather than nourishing the family or resettling the family in a more secure area.

Comparisons among Ethnic Groups

Hundreds of addicts from diverse ethnic groups appeared at the National Detoxification Center in Vientiane (the capital city) seeking treatment for narcotic addiction. This allowed demographic and clinical comparisons to be made among a large number of ethnic groups including those native to Laos (Lao, Hmong, or Meo, and other ethnic groups), expatriate groups who had been resident in Laos for decades or even generations (the Chinese and Vietnamese), more transient expatriate Asians (the Thai and Indian-Pakistanis), and expatriate Caucasians from Europe and North America. A comparison between a group of Hmong patient-addicts from this sample and Hmong addicts from previous nonpatient samples indicated that the addicts in the patient sample were similar to addicts at large in the population for most demographic and clinical variables (18).

The 81 Hmong addict-patients differed from other addict-patients in several aspects. They were about a decade younger (average age of 39.2 years with a standard deviation of 9.4 years). They had the highest proportion of female addicts, with a sex ratio of 2.7 men to every one woman. All were using opium; none were addicted to heroin. And their age at the time of first becoming addicted to narcotics was about a decade younger than other addicts (mean age of 27.6 years with a standard deviation of 9.3 years). These differences were most likely accounted for by the fact that the Hmong were opium poppy farmers; opium was their primary cash crop and most Hmong families raised it. Opium was thus available in virtually all Hmong homes. Since most Hmong were rural-dwelling peoples, far removed from the urban opium dens, most opium usage occurred within the home. Hmong were therefore exposed to opium at an early age, and women were more exposed to its usage than women among other ethnic groups. It is of interest that the duration of addiction among Hmong patients seeking treatment was about the same as those from other ethnic groups, indicating that the duration of addiction was a more critical variable in determining motivation for admission than were other variables, such as age.

An unexpected finding at the treatment facility was that about 60 percent of the addicts seeking treatment were ethnic Lao (321 out of a total 532 addicts). The literature (3), as well as repeated comments by many Lao officials, had indicated that most addicts in Laos were not ethnic Lao, but ethnic Hmong and Chinese. However, Lao addicts came from literally every province in the country and from all social classes (including the elite) in order to seek treatment. It was even more surprising to learn that opium addicts were to be found among the children and wives of the elite (including generals, police colonels, and former ministers), and even in the King's household. Lao addicts had comprised a "hidden" population. (This "hidden" aspect has been borne out by my earlier survey among 40 nonpatient addicts, among whom only nine Lao addicts were encountered [10].) This sample of Lao addicts contained relatively few females (only 19 out of 321, or six percent of the total Lao group). In addition, a recent outbreak of heroin usage was noted among the Lao addicts; 38 subjects (11 percent of the total 321 Lao addicts)—all men and all from the Vientiane area—were using heroin (16).

Expatriate Asian addicts (including the Vietnamese, Chinese, Indian-Pakistanis, and Thai) were like the ethnic Lao addicts in most regards. That is, their current age and the age at which they became addicted were similar to the Lao, there were relatively fewer women among them, and a small percentage of them were using heroin. Like the Lao and Hmong, about 90 percent were married, most were currently living with their families, and a vast majority of them were currently employed at some occupation. Unlike the Lao and the Hmong, however, most of them lived in towns and relatively few of them were peasant farmers (17).

Another unexpected phenomena was the frequency with which "world traveler" addicts from Europe and the United States presented to the National Detoxification Center for treatment. This was unexpected because the staff of the center were Lao, and the Lao language was the lingua franca spoken at the center (though a few members could speak some limited French and English). Over a period of 30 months, 130 such addicts came for treatment. Data obtained from 56 of them indicated that they were predominantly young (mean age of 26.1 years, standard deviation of 6.3 years). About 70 percent of them (39 out of 56) were single and another 9 percent were divorced (5 out of 56). About 60 percent were living alone (33 out of 56), and most were unemployed indigents or tourists. Approximately a fifth of them (11 out of 56) were female. The majority were using heroin (46 out of 56), and 27 of these were using it by injection while the remainder took it by smoking or sniffing it (19). They had been addicted a relatively short time compared to the Asian addicts.

Treatment Acceptance and Efficacy

Treatment for opium addiction was not a new concept to the people of Laos. A variety of folk treatment methods were known (12). While none of the traditional treatment modalities were noted for their efficacy, they were, nonetheless, often used by addicts motivated by increasing problems to abandon their addictive behavior—and occasional cases of successful outcomes did occur.

In early 1971 the Ministry of Welfare in Laos actually funded one traditional treatment modality, that of "cold turkey" withdrawal under the supervision of Buddhist monks at a temple. Initially large numbers of addicts took advantage of this treatment modality (in total, over 2,000 of them). However, the discomfort attendant on the treatment and the significant mortality gradually became known around the country, and by 1973 few addicts were seeking this form of treatment.

The National Detoxification Center in Vientiane—established by the Ministry of Health in late 1972— provided methadone detoxification, in addition to care for associated medical problems. From the day it opened, addicts sought admission to the facility in large numbers. Moreover, a wide diversity of ethnic groups sought treatment at the facility, including groups with a traditional distrust of ethnic Lao (such as the Hmong) and even Americans and Europeans who tended not to use indigenous health care institutions. About 2,000 addicts were treated in the 30 months between September 1972, and March 1975. The occupancy rate at the treatment facility ran well over 90 percent when averaged for the year, and addicts voluntarily came from every corner of the country at their own expense in order to seek treatment (17, 20). The readmission rate within 365 days of discharge was 17.6 percent during the first 12 months of operation. Most readmissions (79 percent of them) were ethnic Lao. Those readmitted were younger and more likely to be using heroin than patients not readmitted.

A follow-up study of patients from the National Detoxification Center was done in 1974. A representative sample of 25 patients was chosen from Vientiane and Xieng Khouang provinces, areas where opium had become less available and more expensive than previously. At a one year follow-up, 16 of these patients (64 percent of the total) were still entirely abstinent from opium. The remaining nine (i.e., 36 percent) had resumed opium usage; but their mean daily cost of opium at one year post-treatment was less than what it had been prior to treatment (U.S. $1.05 per day at the time of admission and U.S. $0.38 per day at the time of follow-up). Another eight addicts were followed up in the Houa Khong province, an area within the Golden Triangle where opium was abundant and inexpensive. All of these addicts had been readdicted within one year and were using amounts similar to what they had been using before treatment. An analysis of the factors that favored abstinence at one year included the following:

1. Detoxification of all or most addicts within a given village or neighborhood at the same time.

2. Satisfactory withdrawal treatment so that the patient was reasonably comfortable at the time of discharge.

3. Amelioration of associated medical problems.

4. Decreased availability and increased cost of narcotic substances.

5. Continued contact with a supportive person interested in the patient's welfare, such as the village chief, village health worker, missionary, or nearby medical facility.

6. Employment, marriage, and residence within a family.

DISCUSSION

Research of opium addiction over the last decade in Laos indicates that some stereotypes regarding Indochinese addicts contain grains of truth. For example, opium usage was not so inherently euphorigenic that one or a few episodes of opiate intoxication inevitably led to chronic addiction in all individuals. Furthermore, some individuals could engage in episodic usage over years or even decades without becoming addicted. And some addicts were able to "control" their addiction for long periods so that biomedical, family, and social problems were kept at a minimum.

Other aspects of the stereotypes did not hold true. Use of opium did comprise a risk for the subsequent development of addiction, especially if one or more of the following factors were present: a family history of opium addiction; association with addicted friends or prolonged isolation from ethnic peers; chronic illness with pain, dysphoria, cough, or diarrhea. In such instances, full-blown narcotic addiction could readily take root within days or a few weeks.

Addiction in Laos gave rise to many of the same problems that clinicians note with alcoholism or narcotic addiction in the United States or elsewhere. These included a variety of biomedical, economic, and family problems. Deprived of legal access to abundant inexpensive opium, the addiction syndrome gave rise to the same kinds of social problems that one can observe in New York City, including criminality, corruption of the police, substitution of heroin for opium, and the use of the injection route of administration in order to conserve heroin.

In summary, these data have guided the government of Laos in the treatment of addicts and formation of social policies regarding narcotic addicts. Moreover, they have added a small increment to our understanding of the narcotic addiction syndrome, and of the sociocultural factors affecting the development and course of the syndrome.

REFERENCES

1. Young, G. Hill tribes of northern Thailand. Bangkok: Siam Society, 1961.
2. Srisavasi, B.C. Hill tribes of Siam. Bangkok: Bomrung Nukoulit Press, 1953.
3. LaBar, F., and Suddard, A. Laos, its people, its society, its culture. New Haven Conn.: Human Relations Area Files Press, 1960.
4. Park, W.H. Opinions of 100 physicians on the use of opium in China. Shanghai: American Presbyterian Mission Press, 1899.
5. Singer, K. The choice of intoxicant among the Chinese. *Brit. J. Addictions,*

   69: 257–268, 1974.
6. Hahn, E. The big smoke. *The New Yorker*, pp. 35–43, February 15, 1969.
7. Howard, H. *Ten Weeks with Chinese Bandits*. London: John Lane The Bodley Head, 1927).
8. Westermeyer, J. The use of alcohol and opium by two ethnic groups in Laos, *Transcult. Psychiat. Rev.*, 6: 148–151,1969.
9. Westermeyer, J. Use of alcohol and opium by the Meo of Laos. *Amer. J. Psychiat.*, 127: 1019–1023, 1971.
10. Westermeyer, J. Opium smoking in Laos: A survey of 40 addicts. *Amer. J. Psychiat.*, 131: 165–170, 1974.
11. Westermeyer, J. Opium dens: A social resource for addicts in Laos, *Arch. Gen. Psychiat.*, 31: 237–240, 1974.
12. Westermeyer, J. Folk treatments for opium addiction in Laos. *Brit. J. Addictions*, 68: 345–349, 1973.
13. Westermeyer, J., and Hausman, W. Mental health consultation with government agencies: A comparison of two cases. *Soc. Psychiat.*, 9: 137–141, 1974.
14. Westermeyer, J., and Hausman W. Cross-cultural consultation for mental health planning. *Internat. J. Soc. Psychiat.*, 20: 34–38, 1974.
15. Westermeyer, J. The pro-heroin effects of anti-opium laws, *Arch. Gen. Psychiat.*, vol. 33: 1135–1139, 1976.
16. Westermeyer, J. A "hidden" addict population in Asia: The Lao. (Unpublished.)
17. Westermeyer, J., and Soudaly, C. An addiction treatment program in Laos: The first year's experience. (Unpublished.)
18. Westermeyer, J., and Peng, G. Two sampling techniques among Hmong opium addicts: A comparison and critique. *British Journal of Addiction*. (In press.)
19. Westermeyer, J., and Berger, L. A study of "stay-at-home" versus "world-traveler" addicts. (In preparation.)
20. Porter, J. Drug addiction in Laos. *Asia Magazine*, 14(6): 12–14, 1974.

Part IV
THE FUTURE OF
CULTURAL PSYCHIATRY

Introduction

I am not sure who first coined the phrase "cultural psychiatry," but it appears to be an older term than cross-cultural psychiatry or transcultural psychiatry. I prefer it to the latter terms because "cross-cultural" refers to a methodology (albeit one of the most important methodologies for studying culture), while "transcultural" has an exotic flavor.

Freud and his immediate followers wrote about culture but never developed a cultural psychiatry. Rather, they attempted to use their techniques and concepts to understand culture. It has been only recently that some analysts have attempted to understand psychiatry by adding the cultural dimensions, e.g., Robert Levy and Robert LeVine.

Joe Yamamoto's essay illustrates how a Western psychiatric approach *must* be modified if it is to be helpful to patients from an

205

Asian culture. Yamamoto has studied the effects of ethnocentrism in psychiatry extensively. His essay represents the accumulated wisdom of years of experience and study. Parenthetically, I have just completed reading *The Makioka Sisters,* a classic novel by the fine twentieth-century Japanese writer, Yunichero Tanizaki. The exquisite portrayal of Japanese family life in this novel helped me appreciate many of the statements in Yamamoto's essay. I firmly believe that one useful method of understanding a culture is to read novels about that culture. Translations of many great Japanese novels are readily available. It should be noted also that the theoretical foundation for modern community psychiatry owes much to a study of behavior in American internment camps for Japanese-Americans during World War II. I refer, of course, to Alexander Leighton's *The Governing of Men.*

E. Mansell Pattison's lengthy and scholarly essay on social system therapy was originally presented at the Annual Conference of the American Group Psychotherapy Association in Boston in February, 1976. Pattison is a Renaissance figure of current psychiatry. His productivity is breathtaking and his interests diverse. His genius lies in providing new directions for psychiatry and his present essay is no exception. He has synthesized a vast literature from several disciplines and has presented a clear rationale for psychiatric involvement with the patient and significant others in the patients' psychosocial network. Pattison's essay presents psychiatry with a broad new perspective. I predict that it will stimulate an extensive range of psychiatric research. Personally, it has led me to embark on a series of studies that deal with the degree of cognitive sharing among members of a psychosocial network. A high degree of cognitive sharing in relevant domains, for example, may prove to be a prerequisite for enhancing the therapeutic effectiveness of a network. Pattison has firmly taken the sometimes nebulous concept of "social system" and placed it into a utilitarian framework.

This section concludes with John and Mary Schwab's thoughtful historical overview of the development of Western cultural psychiatry. The authors clearly demonstrate that many notable psychiatrists have struggled to incorporate the cultural dimension into their psychiatric perspective. They point out that the scientific concept of culture has developed in roughly the same time-frame in which modern psychiatry has developed. They correctly note that "Any view of a mentally ill person that does not place him in a cultural perspective is bound to be myopic." They cite several significant examples of areas in which psychiatrists could profit from a cultural approach—modern epidemics, violent events of adolescence, acculturation, problems of individuals and groups, and the comingling of subcultural groups in urban areas. The Schwabs clearly present a strong case for the inclusion of the cultural dimension in psychiatric thinking.

In their totality these essays demonstrate that cultural psychiatry is not merely an exotic area but that it is significant for understanding and for effectively helping *all* people from the most "primitive" to the most "complex." We are all conceived and born in a culture, we grow up and prosper in a culture, and eventually we die in a culture. *All* psychiatric syndromes are culture-bound even though, as may be the case with some schizophrenias, there may be some universal components to psychopathology. By adding the cultural dimension to our understanding of mental health and illness, we are bound to become wiser, more compassionate, and more effective healers. Cultural psychiatry does not promise a millenium, but it does promise to complement and to enhance biological and psychological psychiatry. The concept of culture is complex and the meaningful study of culture is difficult, but cultural psychiatry is an idea whose time has finally arrived.

16

An Asian View of
The Future of Cultural Psychiatry

JOE YAMAMOTO

We are in an era of cultural pluralism. Cultural psychiatry needs to reassess our culture-bound conceptions and premises. It is important that human behavior be related to its current and past culture, instead of assuming that an American melting pot is a homogenized standard. Just as a psychiatrist must evaluate a patient's background, problems, requests, and objectives, we must also consider evaluations of a culture from a psychiatric viewpoint. I believe that there are several ways to approach this. I will approach it via clinical evaluation of Asian patients and a discussion of the cultural derivation of specific Japanese therapeutic methods.

EVALUATION OF PATIENTS

American evaluation of patients is too often a one-dimensional focus on the individual. Some American psychiatrists have emphasized family therapy, but most are biased toward individual treatment. Even in group therapy, the individual enters without reference to his real groups, family, kinfolk, relationships, and friends. The picture in the therapist's mind is of the rugged individualist fending for himself, struggling for individual success, instead of cooperation.

It is apparent that this does not fit the common conception of interpersonal relationships in Asian countries. In Asia the individual is not the primary unit, it is the family (1–4). The family unit is headed by the patriarch. In contrast to our egalitarian values, the relationships are vertical (5). This family picture of relationships extends to the patient and doctor relationship. The doctor is like the patriarch and is an authority figure. This was vividly demonstrated to me during a visit to Tokyo where I observed the interactions between the doctor and patient. In Japan, one can evaluate the social status of individuals by observing how one bows to the other. The doctor (the *Sensei*) almost imperceptibly tilted his head as the patient formally bowed, not only his head, but his entire trunk.

This vignette about bowing behavior is part of a culturally relevant interaction and one aspect of the conception of the doctor-patient role. I believe this description of the bows is symbolic of the doctor's authoritarian role.

The popular American notion of the therapist as a relatively neutral, nonjudgmental, noncritical person would seem alien in Asian cultures. Indeed, the conception of the therapist as a passive, inactive, non-directive facilitator of the patient's verbalization would be contrary to the patient's expectations (6).

We must also remember that the family is much more often involved in decision making. Thus, the therapeutic contract between the physician and the patient as viewed by Ralph Greenson (7), for example, would only be possible with the minority of Asian patients. Usually the agreement would have to be between the doctor and the family.

The diagnoses have to be sensitive to the Asian culture. For example, in the formal examination, patients can pull themselves together and behave as their culture demands (8). Even psychotic patients may behave politely and appropriately. Because of this and for other diagnostic reasons, it is appropriate to get collateral history from relatives and friends. In Asia there is a bias against psychiatry and against the mentally ill, so the patients may be sick longer and more seriously before the psychiatrist sees them. Indeed, in Japan in the last decade the number of hospitalized patients has grown almost geometrically so that with approximately half of the population of the United States, they have twice as many hospitalized psychiatric patients

—suggesting that Japanese psychiatry had advanced beyond us in hospital care (9). Yet Japanese patients suffer from these advances of psychiatry, for the profession has all too efficiently arranged for hospital treatment, instead of more appropriate treatment in the community. Another aspect of this situation is the fact that National Health Insurance covers mainly hospital care and only minimally offers any outpatient coverage.

Finally, another example concerning cultural factors which must be considered for appropriate diagnosis is the evaluation of dependency versus independence. In Japan, the average person has been socialized to be a part of an interdependent family group (10). Thus, the picture in the American psychiatrist's mind of the idealized rugged individual does not apply in Asia, or to Asian-Americans. An Asian patient may be chronologically adult, but still closely related to his parents and siblings as a child and member of the family unit—this would be the usual pattern of interdependence. The parents expect that the children will nourish, support, and take care of them when they become old. It would be an error to assume that such behavior is due to psychopathological dependency such as that in a passive-dependent personality. There are mutual concerns, obligations, and responsibilities within the family.

TREATMENT OF ASIANS

More accurate cultural diagnosis should be matched by culturally sensitive treatment. The therapist should understand the importance of Asian familism. In addition, he should know the importance of close family ties. For example, Japanese families dine together, work together, bathe together, and sleep together. Togetherness is a lifelong process. The traditional Japanese hospital provides for the family representative to stay at the hospital, share the room, and prepare the meals. There is great concern about continuing the family. Marriages are often still arranged. The bride joins the groom's family (one important exception is when the bride's family has no male heir—then the groom may agree to be a *Yoshi* and assume the bride's surname to continue the family). When possible the newlyweds share space in the parental home.

Because of these factors, the family must much more often be seen, they must be engaged in the treatment program and directed toward therapeutic goals. The father may be too busy at work to actively participate, but the mother, grandparents, and/or siblings may be actively involved. The family can be mobilized to be a sustaining, helping group to augment the therapy of the individual.

Of course there are situations where the approach must vary. There may be patients, for example, who are threatened by family prohibitions. One example would be the choice of an unapproved vocational goal. Should career choice be a part of the intrafamily conflict, then separate sessions with parents may be indicated in order to evaluate the extent of their rigidity versus their desires. All of these considerations should lead to a much more flexible conception of therapy, often including family members, and with the psychotherapist often directing the entire family unit toward improved patient well-being.

JAPANESE INTROSPECTIVE THERAPIES

In Japan various approaches to the treatment of neurotic and personality problems have developed. Although they are not the predominant methods of treatment, that is to say, practiced by a majority of psychiatrists and other therapists, I believe it is important to thoroughly learn what we can from these different approaches. There are two forms of therapy that include introspection and specific instructions by the doctor.

Morita Therapy

Morita Therapy was devised by Dr. S. Morita. The original method was to place the patient in isolation for a week or two and follow this with progressive activity. The aim was not symptomatic relief, but improved functioning. To quote David Reynolds (11):

> Nevertheless, he is to direct his attention to getting the job done. He has been warned that the joy [of doing the work] would pass, too, that feelings are changeable "like the Japanese sky." Life is not to be based on feelings but on productive activity. One can build a sense of self-worth on what he has accomplished for others.
>
> The goal of therapy thereafter is to so immerse the patient in the needs of the moment so that he loses awareness of the symptoms, the nagging anxiety, the unappeasable pain. To sit and reflect on it only exaggerates it and inflates its effect on his consciousness.

According to Reynolds, the Morita therapist makes it clear to the patients that they are responsible for what they do, that they have direct control over their behavior. This is in contrast to the patient's condition, impulses, feelings, which are not directly under the patient's control. Along with the instructions by the doctor, there is an emphasis on being aware of what is going on from moment to moment, and the patient is requested to keep a diary which he then discusses with the doctor. The goal of this introspection is to focus on external reality rather than on inner feelings, symptoms, and problems. Finally, as a part of the terminal phase of hospitalization, there are group discussions and the patient may subsequently join the Morita Group as an outpatient.

Naikan Therapy

In Naikan Therapy, the patient or subject is instructed to sit in a small, enclosed, boothlike area. This therapy method was initiated with prisoners in jail who were instructed to face a blank wall in the cell. The doctor or therapist instructs the subject to think about his past life in three-year periods, beginning with the period from birth to age three, three to age six, etc. During the introspection, he is instructed to see what he can recall concerning his past relationships with people—his mother, father, siblings, teachers, wife, employers, and significant others. The recollections are to focus on: (1) what he received from that person (in terms of objects, services, acts of kindness, etc.), (2) what he returned to that person, and (3) what troubles, inconveniences, deceit, pettiness, and so forth he was responsible for in relation to that person. The ideal is to spend about 20 percent of one's meditation time on each of the first two themes and 60 percent on the third theme. The process may take a week or longer of introspection from early morning until bedtime. The therapist sees the subject every hour or two to check on the progress. The therapist wants to make sure that the subject is recalling the proper memories and the feelings of obligations expected in the Japanese culture.

Discussion

Both Morita and Naikan Therapy are rooted in the Japanese culture. They share several common features: (1) introspection, (2) directions about what to think about, (3) expectations of behavior to suit the Japanese values, and (4) the objective of a person who fits into the Japanese way of life including having filial piety, an achievement orientation, and a strong sense of obligations and responsibility.

Though these therapies have different bases, they do spring from Japan's Buddhist teachings and past Chinese Confucian influences. Because they are so rooted, the end result is a person who will fit into a prescribed pattern of living in Japan's highly structured and vertical society.

SUMMARY

I have chosen to discuss the diagnosis of Asian patients and culturally relevant treatment methods to point out the need in the future of a culturally pluralistic psychiatrist. We in the field of cultural psychiatry must be fully aware of the European bases of American psychiatry and be able to see the blind spots inherent in this tradition. The evaluation of the introspective therapies points out how Japanese values may shape the therapeutic process and objectives. The hoped-for end product is a person who can fit into the family and society in an acceptable and positive manner. These issues are also important for those who train foreign psychiatrists who plan to return to their homeland. In this instance, the education and training should be tailored to the needs.

The future of cultural psychiatry lies in an ever-broadening and pluralistic view of human behavior. We cannot remain with the conception of the Victorian Viennese society, or with the American technological views of the behaviorist. We must add the important factor of culture and how this determines our behavior, especially when we evaluate Americans from Asian and other cultures that differ from the stereotype of American middle-class society.

REFERENCES

1. Hahn, D. Maturity in Korea and America. In: *Transcultural Research in Mental Health,* ed. W.P. Lebra. Honolulu: University Press of Hawaii, 1972.
2. Tung, T-M. The family and the management of mental health problems in Viet Nam. In: *Transcultural Research in Mental Health,* ed. W.P. Lebra. Honolulu: University Press of Hawaii.
3. Yamamoto, K. A Comparative study of patienthood in Japanese and American mental hospitals. In: *Transcultural Research in Mental Health,* ed. W.P. Lebra. Honolulu: University Press of Hawaii, 1972.
4. Yeh, E-K. Paranoid manifestations among Chinese students studying abroad. In: *Transcultural Research in Mental Health,* ed. W.P. Lebra. Honolulu: University Press of Hawaii, 1972.
5. Nakane, C. *Japanese Society.* Berkeley: University of California Press, 1970.
6. Tseng, W-S. et al. Suggestions for intercultural psychotherapy. In: *People and Cultures in Hawaii,* ed. W-S Tseng, J.F. McDermott, T.W. Maretzki, and W. Thomas. Honolulu: University Press of Hawaii, 1974.
7. Greenson, R. The Technique and Practice of Psychoanalysis, Volume I, International University Press, Inc., New York, 1967.
8. Yamamoto, J. Asian psychiatric research priorities. Presented at the

Asian American Mental Health Research Center, La Jolla, California, 1976.

9. Yamamoto, J. et al. Four opinions of psychiatry in Japan. *Clin. Psychiat. Seishin Igaku* (Tokyo), 16: 588–601, 1974.

10. Doi, T. *The Anatomy of Dependence*. Tokyo: *Kodansha International*, 1973.

11. Reynolds, D. *The Quiet Therapies*. (in press.)

17

A Theoretical-Empirical Base For Social System Therapy

E. MANSELL PATTISON, M.D.

This chapter is an attempt to generate formal statements that may serve as a conceptual and theoretical base for the development of clinical methods of mental health treatment that focus on social system interventions.

For some years there has been growing recognition that emotional disorder, in part, has its roots in the social milieu of the individual. Similarly, there have been numerous clinical experiments with treatment methods which have moved into interventions with larger and more complex social systems in which the individual patient is embedded. This might be termed a social psychology of mental illness and treatment.

The problem to this point has been that the theory and data on the social psychology of mental illness have been developed on a macrosystem level, which does not provide a substantial link between the macroprocesses and the individual. On the other hand, the treatment methods, which might be termed applied social psychology, have been developed on the basis of ad hoc clinical empiricism, with no strong link to a scientific base of theory and experimental data. We thus end up with an elegant macrotheory of social psychology and an exciting array of clinical ventures, without a substantial relationship.

I have therefore set out to develop a data base that may establish a middle-range set of concepts and theory linking macrosocial process with individual process. To do so, I shall review data from family therapy, community psychiatry, family sociology, and network analysis in social anthropology. I shall then set forth several theoretical constructs that lead to a clinical typology for social system methods of treatment.

CLINICAL EXTENSIONS OF FAMILY THERAPY

The field of family therapy has grown to a position of major theoretical dominance in the past decade. In his 1974 presidential address, John Spiegel (1) terms family therapy the major organizing concept for psychotherapy of the future. Yet the development of the theory and technique of family therapy has been based primarily on clinical experience with "nuclear" families. By nuclear family, I mean a married couple and their children who have not attained legal majority. It is assumed that this is the "typical" American family structure, for the literature on family therapy focuses almost exclusively on the intact nuclear family. I shall not review that literature.

However, the importance of a larger concept of family as a social system was presented in 1962 by Norman W. Bell (2). He reported that the extended social kinship system was critical to the function of the nuclear family. Bell observed that "well" families had achieved satisfying relations with family kin who provided a major psychosocial resource to the family, whereas "sick" families lived in obvious conflict with their social kin system. He noted that sick families used extended kin in a variety of pathological ways: (1) to reinforce family defenses, (2) as a stimuli for conflict, (3) as a screen for projection of nuclear family conflict, and (4) as competing objects for support.

The first clinical experiment with a *system* of therapy beyond the nuclear family was probably the development of group psychotherapy for married couples, in which four or five nuclear couples are treated in a group (3). The second step was the introduction of multiple family therapy, in which four or five nuclear families are treated in a large group (4–6). The technique of multiple family therapy has been described as one in which the family learns how to operate as a family system within a larger system. One pioneer of this method, H. Peter Laquer (7), describes this as a "system" therapy.

A third step occurred as a result of the conduct of family therapy in the home of the nuclear family (8–10). Here family therapists reported that friends, relatives, and neighbors would occasionally be included in the family sessions because of happenstance or invitation by the family, or they might even be specifically invited into the family by the therapist because the "extra-familial" person seemed to play an important role in the dynamics of the family (11–14). In sum, these rather casual clinical experiences began to demonstrate the importance of other persons in the psychodynamic function of the nuclear family.

A fourth step was the formalization of family therapy groups to include not only the nuclear family, but also persons related either by blood, marriage, friendship, neighboring residence, or work association (15–34). The clinical pioneers in this effort have reported their work as an attempt to collect, organize, and utilize the total social network of the identified patient. The method, thus far, has been termed "network" therapy, "ecological systems" therapy, and "case-linking."

Meanwhile, there has been some explicit recognition by family therapists that the typical nuclear family is not representative of all existent family structures. For example, Sager et al. (35) conclude their work on black family therapy by observing: "the traditional definition of family that guides acceptance into a family clinic must be expanded. The notion of a legally bound adult couple or of the primacy of the nuclear family over other kinship ties is not germane... family has to be redefined.... the therapist frequently works with only fragments of the nuclear or extended family, or with combinations [of relationships]."

Another example is the seminal work of Minuchin and his colleagues (36, 37). In the book *Families of the Slums* (36), they found that slum families often consisted of various fragments of nuclear families and/or extended kinship systems involving both relatives, friends, and neighbors. Because of these observations, Minuchin proposed a more crisis-oriented, reality-based style of family therapy that involved the actual psychosocial family unit, which was not an intact nuclear family.

In brief, family therapists have come to recognize that the basic social unit may not be the nuclear family, or even a family kinship per se, but a collage of persons related in an intimate psychosocial kinship network (38–41).

CONTEMPORARY FAMILY SOCIOLOGY

A major topic of Western sociology has been the changing structure and function of the family. Up to 1945, the major proposition advanced was that the traditional extended family kinship system was gradually disappearing. In place of the extended family was the so-called isolated nuclear family. Two factors, rapid industrialization and a shift to urbanization, were thought to coalesce in the "nuclearization" of families. This trend was viewed with some alarm by family sociologists (42–44). It was apparent that the extended kinship system had provided two major resources for individual and family sustenance. One resource was *affective* support, that is, emotional involvement, personal interest, and psychological support. The other resource was *instrumental* support, that is, the supply of money, food, clothes, and assistance in living and work tasks. The loss of the extended family system that occurred when young couples moved to the city and assumed new jobs different from their agrarian small-town parentage was thought to represent a major loss of affective and instrumental support to the young nuclear family. Some theorists, such as Talcott Parsons (45), concluded that the nuclear family could not survive as a stable family form because it lacked the affective and instrumental resources of the extended kinship. It was hoped that voluntary associations would replace the kinship associations system, although there was little data to support such a hope for new kinships.

A number of studies since 1950 have called into question this industrial-urban nuclearization hypothesis. Komarevsky (46) reported that urban working class families did not associate in voluntary groups, but did retain high levels of socialization with their blood kinship systems. Dotson (74) replicated this finding with further data on high social activity in the kinship system. By 1968 Adams (42, 48) had accumulated a large-enough repertoire of research studies to firmly conclude that at least among the working-class urban families of America the extended kinship system of family structure was not only present, but was the dominant family structure of the urban working class.

But what of the middle-class and upper-class nuclear families that had become the sociological prototype of the new American family? Here again the stereotype does not hold. In 1957 Elizabeth Bott (49, 50) reported that middle-class couples did not live in isolation but formed coalitions with other middle-class couples in a new network of social kinship. In 1959 Sussman (44) reported that "many neolocal nuclear families are closely related within a matrix of mutual assistance and activity which results in a kin related family system." Similarly, in 1967 Herbert Gans (51, 52) found that suburban communities rapidly organized into quasi-family kinship groups that assumed both the affective and instrumental activities of the typical extended kinship structure.

I cannot adequately summarize this extensive family sociology literature, save to note its existence (53–62). The major findings are that there are four major types of family structure in the United States:

1. The traditional extended family that is an interdependent social and economic unit, each nuclear subfamily living in geographic proximity and depending upon the extended kin for major affective and instrumental resources.

2. The dissolving or weak family in which most kin functions have been taken over by large-scale formal organizations, leaving the nuclear family with few resources and few innate coping abilities.

3. The isolated nuclear family, which retains fewer essential functions, but whose functions are concentrated in the family and are maintained with stability, although often at the expenditure of great effort to maintain family cohesion.

4. The modified extended family structure consisting of a coalition of nuclear families in a state of partial dependence.

On a clinical basis, I suggest that the Type 1 traditional extended family is typical of the American working class, and of the very rich upper class. The Type 2 weak-dissolving family is found in the slums and ghettos. The Type 3 isolated nuclear family is found in upwardly mobile and geographically mobile middle-class families. This type family may be overrepresented in clinical family-treatment clinics because it is so vulnerable to stress. In contrast, the Type 4 modified kinship family is the more usual middle-class and upper-middle-class family that makes a successful life adaptation.

In summary, these data suggest that the American family still retains a significant extended kinship system, even in the face of industrialization and urbanization. Further, those working-class and middle-class families that have lost their blood-marriage kinship system, actively re-create a kinship system comprised of the *functional kin*—a friend, neighbor, associate kin system.

EXPERIMENTS IN COMMUNITY PSYCHIATRY

One of the major theorems of community psychiatry is that the individual is a social creature (27, 28, 63, 64). Thus his well-being and capacity to cope with life stress is dependent upon the adequacy of the social-support structures in his life (65, 66). At a more middle-range of theory, it is proposed by several researchers (67–72) that the small intimate social groups of which a person is a member serve to support and sustain effective everyday life and effectively respond to crisis (73–75).

These concepts have been implemented in clinical practice in several ways. First is the assessment of social-support relations at the time of initial evaluation, with treatment plans developed on the basis of these social resources. Treatment then proceeds through the linking of the client to his social resources (17–19, 22, 76–78). Second, attempts have been made to mobilize natural resources within the community to respond to people in stress so that contact with formal mental health services is averted (79, 80). Third, clinicians have mobilized neighborhoods to form mutual support groups (81–83). Finally, others have sought to engage in preventive work through the mobilization of non-treatment crisis support among community members (84–88).

In all of these instances, there is explicit recognition that effective mental health intervention must go beyond the identified patient, and must link the patient to his actual or potential community social-support resources. It is recognized that mental health rehabilitation may not reside primarily in the therapist treating the patient, but rather in mobilizing an effective social network of intervention and rehabilitation. Researchers (89–93) working from the view of ecological psychology have devised methods to map participation in community networks. Their findings are similar to those of the clinicians cited: that different groups of alienated persons have low community participation, while alienation is reduced through activation of community interactions (94).

NETWORK ANALYSIS IN SOCIAL ANTHROPOLOGY

During the past 20 years, there has been a slow but steady development in social anthropology of the structure and function of social networks. These anthropologists hold that the concentration on cultural rules, belief systems, and groups in the formal theory of anthropology has failed to grasp the function of the individual. Indeed, classical anthropology has seen social networks as the residual of cultural process, rather than as the creator of cultural process. This new anthropological orientation seeks to bring to the foreground a social analysis of the internal process and inherent dynamics in relations between inter-dependent human beings. Network analysis in anthropology is then an attempt to define the structure and function of the primary social relations of the individual, as well as derivative relations. This work, primarily by European social anthropologists, has shown how effective analysis of social networks can be constructed (95–97).

There are two ways to look at social networks. First there is the *objective* network. This is a network arbitrarily defined by the specific criterion that motivates the analysis. For instance, we may wish to examine the objective family network, a work network, a rumor network, a political network, a clinic or day-care treatment network, etc. In other words, we define the objective frame-reference, and then look in the community to see who exists in that objective frame. The community is a tapestry woven of many threads of relationships. In an objective network analysis, we define the specific thread of relationships and follow that thread throughout the community. This is the pattern of analysis used in most community-psychiatry projects of network construction. The clinician specifies the clinical task he wishes to accomplish, identifies the set of relations he wishes to utilize or construct, and then organizes or convenes that objective network. In sum, *we define the objective network by the social purpose we seek.*

The second kind of network is the subjective network. This is a phenomenological world of relationships as defined and experienced by the individual. The *subjective network can only be defined by the individual.* The subjective network of the individual overlaps many different objective networks, such as family, work, recreation, etc. The objective network of a person's extended family may include spouse, children, grandparents, in-laws, aunts, uncles, and cousins. Yet the same person's psychosocial kinship system—his subjective network—may not include most of these objective kin, but may include his close family, good neighbors, best friends, and close work and recreational associates. As we shall see, it is important to consider both objective and subjective network analysis as a framework for clinical intervention.

The second aspect of network analysis is the zones of relationships. Boissevain (95) points out that a person may have contact with over 1,500 people in his life interactions, yet this vast array of people is not uniformly related to the person, rather they are arranged in zones of intimacy, importance, and basis of relationship. A first-order zone contains the person's nuclear family, with whom there is regular contact, intimate relationship, and high degrees of instrumental and affective exchange. The second-order zone comprises close friends, neighbors, co-workers, and relatives who are of high significance to the person and with whom there is a high degree of structured and expectable exchange of affective and instrumental resources. The first and second zones comprise what I call the "intimate psychosocial network."

Beyond these two, the third zone consists of persons with whom one has less regular contact, such as distant friends and relatives, or people whom one sees frequently but does not value highly, such as neighbors or co-workers. Here there is a network of *potential relations.* As they make geographic moves, change jobs, or enter different life stages, people may move between these three zones. The third zone

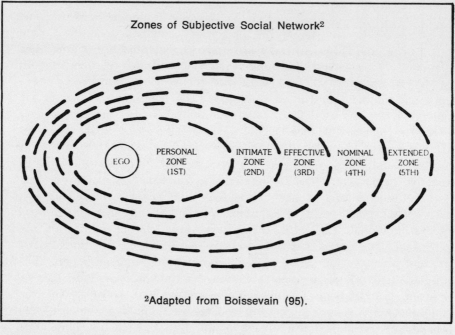

Zones of Subjective Social Network[2]

EGO — PERSONAL ZONE (1ST) — INTIMATE ZONE (2ND) — EFFECTIVE ZONE (3RD) — NOMINAL ZONE (4TH) — EXTENDED ZONE (5TH)

[2]Adapted from Boissevain (95).

1

is important as a recruitment area for mobilizing social resources for the person.

The fourth zone is the so-called *effective zone*. These are people who are strategically important to a person, and therefore relationships are maintained to some degree, so that use can be made of these resources. This zone might include the family doctor, business acquaintances, neighborhood relations, etc. The fifth zone is the *nominal zone* and consists of people known only casually, by reputation, as representatives of agencies or services. Such people would come into relation with the person only if they possessed needed services, resources, or became linked to the individual through intermediaries. Examples might be the minister of a close friend who meets the person through the friend; or a job offer from a manager met through introduction by a mutual colleague.

In Figure 1 the different zones are shown in graphic form, as a representation of the subjective egocentric social network.

Another way of looking at the construction of social networks is

Table 1
Types of Social Networks[a]

Limited Network (set) Any extract of the total network based on some criterion applicable throughout the whole network					Unlimited Network
Personal Set	Categorical Set	Action Set	Role-System Set	Field Set	The social network conceived
Limited to links of one person	Limited to links involving persons of a certain type or category	Limited to links purpose-fully used for a specific end	Limited to links involved in an organized role system or group	Limited to links with a certain con-tent (eco-nomic, polit-ical, etc.)	without application of limit-ing criteria

[a]Adapted from Whitten and Wolfe (98).

presented by Whitten and Wolfe (98). It combines both the objective network and the subjective network. This is shown in Table 1.

Briefly, the *personal set* is the egocentric subjective network. The other types are objective networks. The *categorical set* would be illus-trated by a family network where the category is kinship. An *action set* would be those people linked to accomplish a given social purpose. For example, a mental health team might link school, police, church, and welfare personnel to aid a family. The *role-system set* involves people in specific role relations, such as all personnel in a hospital or office. The relationship is determined by the organizational linkage that spreads rumors through an office or a oommunity, or the common interest of a service or recreational club.

The importance of this is that it clarifies the question of where to begin in constructing a social system for intervention. Much of the clinical work with social systems has been ad hoc with no clear specifica-tion of which type of social network was to be used to define precisely whom one wants to contact in the elaboration of a specific type of social network.

A third network concept has to do with the density or connected-ness of the network. By this I refer to the amount of interaction and relatedness between members of a given network. If we look at the subjective network, it is obvious that most people in the intimate psychosocial network will have some type of ongoing relationships apart from ego. That is, there is a *group* of people who exist in a state of partial interdependence. On the other hand, a field set that comprises a rumor network may consist of linear relations where no one knows more than one other person in the network.

The importance of network density is of significance to the behavior of the network. The more dense a network, the more speedy is communication through multiple channels, the more group consensus on values and desired action, and the more capacity for mobilization for concerted action toward a goal. It is thus important to specify not only the number of people in a network, and the basis of relationship, but also the degree of interconnection that converts the social *network* into a social *group* to greater or lesser degree.

One final issue must be raised—the stability and uniformity of the personal social network. In the rural village setting, the social network is comprised of preponderance of kin. Recent studies on migration to urban settings show that people do reconstitute a new social network of approximately the same size, and that the size of the social network remains relatively constant across various social classes. The one difference in social class, however, is that the lower social classes in urban settings tend to populate their networks with kin and informal neighborhood relations, while upper social classes tend to populate their networks from formal associations and organizations (99–105).

In summary, this work in social anthropology supports the concept that the social network is a basic unit for social analysis, for the social network is the intermediary between the individual and his social sources of behavior. Further, each person participates in multiple social networks. There is no one social network, although the person may only consciously perceive his own egocentric phenomenological network. The social networks shift and change over time; they do not remain fixed. Even the egocentric network shifts. Boissevain (96) reports that in a five-year period, 50 percent of the people in the intimate psychosocial network changed. Thus, network analysis is not a search for a fixed social unit, but rather the definition of a functional social system of relationships.

MENTAL HEALTH AND THE SOCIAL NETWORK

How important is the psychosocial system for the maintenance of mental health, and what is the relation between mental health and one's social network? At this point, we can state that the presumptive evidence is strong, although direct evidence is just beginning to be acquired.

The first line of evidence comes from family sociology, where there is a wealth of data demonstrating that there is a high level of interchange of both instrumental and affective assistance that flows between members of extended kinship and psychosocial kinship social systems. By inference we may conclude that the individuals and nuclear families without such social-support systems are at least highly vulnerable to stress and crisis (106–111).

A more direct line of evidence comes from sociological studies of actual help-seeking behavior. These nonclinical studies repeatedly show that families do turn to their psychosocial network for instrumental and affective assistance without use of formal helping and service agencies. Both Croog et al. (112) and McKinlay (113) found that the psychosocial system is the preferred resource for help even in cases of severe physical illness. Extensive help reliance on the personal psychosocial system is reported by Lebowitz et al. (114), Salloway and Dillon (115), and Young (110, 111).

The above studies show that the psychosocial network is utilized in order to cope effectively with life. But is the psychosocial network critical for effective functioning? In terms of family function there are several pertinent studies. Bell (2) showed that sick and well families have different kinship relationships. Kammeyer and Bolton (116) compared normal families and families seeking psychological treatment. The "sick" families had fewer memberships in voluntary associations, fewer friendships with relatives, and fewer relations living in the same community. Alissi (15) and Feldman and Scherz (107) report the lack of an effective social network in families seeking treatment. When we look at individual function vis-à-vis the social network, we find similar supportive data. Hammer (117) found that ineffective networks correlated with mental hospital admission. Brim (118) reports that personal happiness is related to an intact, effective social network. Finally, the most direct test of the hypothesis is found in the work of Kleiner and Parker (119). They used three measures of psychosocial impairment: history of nervous or mental disorder, a measure of self-esteem, and psychoneurotic symptom score. They then measured the degree of importance of and the degree of alienation of the individual from his family network, friend network, and co-worker network. They found that alienation from each of the three networks was significantly related to all three measures of psychosocial impairment, alienation was cumulatively related to psychosocial impairment, and degree of alienation and impairment varied directly with the importance of the network. Supportive evidence is given by Giovannoni and Billingsley (120). They found that inadequate mothers who demonstrated manifest child neglect had friends and relatives nearby, but the presence of these social resources was not enough. The neglectful mothers were alienated from and did not use their available psychosocial network. I shall present my direct data in support of the hypothesis shortly.

This brief summary indicates that the psychosocial network or system does exist. Second, the psychosocial system exerts both positive and negative sanctions and supports for the nuclear family and for the individual. Third, the psychosocial system is a fundamental social matrix that may be pathological or therapeutic. This evidence supports the contention by Jackson (121) that we must move from the family as primary social group to the larger context of the psychodynamic social system of the individual.

This leads us to a diagnostic focus on the social system. One major book has formulated this approach. In *Kinship and Casework*, Leichter and Mitchell (122) conclude:

> We have argued that family diagnosis must not end with the nuclear family, because the family is no more a closed equilibrium system than is the individual.... Knowledge of the relationships between the family and its external environment are vital ... this knowledge applies to kin, to occupational associates, to friends, and other non-familial relationships.... This unit would differ radically in some of the characteristics of externally impersonal relationships that pertain in group therapy.... A group of kin might be an effective unit of treatment precisely because they are interrelated, and changes in one would have actual relevance for changes in the others ... the possibility that this unit might be effective in some instances is no more far-fetched than the notion that the family rather than the individual is sometimes the appropriate unit of treatment.

The use of extended family kinship groups as the target for evaluation and intervention is also underscored by Mendell et al. (123–125). They suggest a focus on this ongoing social system (124): "When the individual comes to a therapist for help, we assume that he is admitting the failure of his group as an effective milieu in which to find the solution he seeks.... Our data suggest that the individual seeking help frequently approaches the therapist to protest against the ineffectiveness of the group to which he belongs."

Finally, the clinical importance of the psychosocial family system is summarized by the following conclusions of Eugene Litwak (57) (he refers to kinship where he says family):

> ... there are several classes of situations where the trained expert is of little use: in situations which are not uniform and

where the minimal standards set by society are not involved. By contrast, the formal organization might be more effective in uniform situations where high social values are involved. The question arises as to whether the family as a primary group might not be superior to the formal organization in these areas ... the family structure is able to deal more easily with the idiosyncratic event because the family has more continuous contact over many different areas of life than the professional organizations ... the family has speedier channels for transmitting messages that had no prior definition of legitimacy ... it is less likely to have explicit rules on what is and what is not legitimate, it is more likely to consider events which have had no definition. ... In most instances the bureaucratic agency is specifically prevented from acting, by explicit rules which define the area of legitimacy ahead of time. ... The family can define much more uniquely what is to be valued. The number of people who must cooperate are much fewer, and because they are involved in affectional relations, they are most inclined to accept each other's personal definition values.

In sum, we have arrived at a point at which we can state with some certainty that the psychosocial system is a primary unit for clinical diagnosis and clinical intervention.

DEFINITION OF THE PSYCHOSOCIAL KINSHIP SYSTEM

Up to this point, the definition of the psychosocial system has been loosely conceptual. Social psychologists have found that mere blood or marriage affinity does not define meaningful kin relationships, nor does a casual definition of friend, neighbor, or work associate define a significant psychodynamic relationship (126–128). Similarly, the clinical reports cited seem to follow circumstance and serendipity in the collation of psychosocial systems, rather than an empirically based concept of a psychosocial organization. Indeed, the most frequent question is: Who constitutes the psychosocial system?

To answer this question, our research team has developed an empirical instrument, the Pattison Psychosocial Kinship Inventory, to determine the exact nature of the psychosocial system. Our aim is to determine the *psychodynamic* social system that comprises the primary social matrix of the individual. The people in this matrix are related to the individual on the basis of both *interaction* and *valued importance*. The relationships in the matrix are thus determined by social and psychological variables. Further, this social matrix represents the *functional kin group* of the individual. Hence we term this the *psychosocial kinship system*.

Our inventory is based on the empirical social psychology of interpersonal relations (48). Significant interpersonal relations are based on five major variables. First, the relationship has a relatively high degree of *interaction*, whether face-to-face, by telephone, or by letter. In other words, a person invests in those with whom he has contact. Second, the relationship has a strong *emotional intensity*. The degree of investment on others is reflected in the intensity of feeling toward the other. Third, the emotion is generally *positive*. Negative relationships are maintained only when other variables force the maintenance of the relationship, such as a boss or spouse. Fourth, the relationship has an *instrumental base*. That is, the other person is not only held in positive emotional regard, but can be counted on to provide concrete assistance. Fifth, the relationship is *symmetrically reciprocal*. That is, the other person returns the strong positive feeling, and may count on you for instrumental assistance. There is an affective and instrumental quid pro quo.

In the administration of the Pattison Psychosocial Kinship Inventory, we ask the individual to list the *subjectively important* people in his life, under the categories of family, relatives, friends, co-workers, and social organization. We then have the subject rate each person listed according to items on the five variables of interpersonal relations. Finally, the subject draws a sociogram of the social connections that exist between all the people he lists. This produces a social-connectedness ratio, that is, the proportion of people in this social matrix who interact with each other.

Preliminary data, based on this method, have been collected for a normative urban population of 200 subjects, and small populations of neurotic and psychotic subjects. Although complete data will not be reported here, we do wish to present certain salient findings to demonstrate the possible clinical utility of this method of mapping out the psychosocial kinship system.

Our data on normal populations reveal that the healthy person has 20 to 30 persons in his intimate psychosocial network. The relationships are rated positive on all five variables of interpersonal relations. There are typically five or six people in each subgroup of family, relatives, friends, neighbors, and work or social contacts. About half to two-thirds of these people have social relations with each other, so that the social-connectedness ratio is about 60 percent. Friends are the most highly valued members of the network outside of the nuclear family, and are most often sought for affective and instrumental assistance. Significant relations are found in multiple areas of life interaction, and the social matrix is semi-open to other people. In summary, the normal person has a finite primary group of about 25 people who comprise a stable, yet not exclusive, psychosocial system.

How valid are these findings? Our empirical findings bear striking correspondence to a series of mathematical formulations in social anthropology. Killworth and Bernard (129) have recently reported work on the theory of random groups in which they attempt to formulate the parameters for social group function: "In general, then, any individual is a member of several different social systems simultaneously; work, family, or social life, these may or may not be intersecting. Presumably people are able to process all these systems simultaneously precisely because they are never asked to do just that." Killworth and Bernard then estimate that the normal person has 24 to 27 direct personal relationships in life; with four to five subgroups each comprised of five to six persons; all related in a pseudoclosed network. This mathematical formulation is thus almost an exact prediction of the structure of the psychosocial network we have defined through our empirical studies. Additional empirical support is found in the work on social networks by the Dutch anthropologist Boissevain (95). He has mapped personal social networks using a technique similar to ours. His data reveal an average of 30 persons in the intimate social network. Consequently, we feel our description of the primary psychosocial kinship system is a relatively accurate generalization.

For our neurotic population, we find a different pattern. They have 10 to 12 people in their network. The network usually includes significant people who are dead or live far away. Ratings on the interpersonal variables are lower than for normals, and usually contain a number of negative relationships. The network has a social-connectedness ratio around 30 percent. It is as if the neurotic is at the hub of a wheel, with individual relations like spokes that have no interrelationship. In sum, the neurotic has an impoverished psychosocial network that does not provide a supportive psychosocial matrix.

For our psychotic population, a third pattern emerges. These people have only four or five people in their network, usually family. Their interpersonal ratings are uniformly ambivalent and nonreciprocal. Their social-connectedness ratio is 90–100 percent. In other words, the psychotic is caught in an exclusive, small social matrix that binds him and fails to provide a healthy interpersonal matrix.

In Table 2 I have summarized our data. These data unequivocally demonstrate that mental illness is related to the quality of the psycho-

Table 2
Social Networks of Normal, Neurotic, Psychotic Subjects

	Normal	Neurotic	Psychotic
Mean number persons in network	25	15	7
Types of relationships in network	Positive Symmetric	Negative Absent/dead members	Ambivalent Only family or transient members
Network density/connection	60%	30%	90%

social network. Further, an examination of the nature of the relationships in the psychosocial network provides guidelines to plan specific therapeutic interventions. For example, where a person encounters a life crisis with an intact, functional psychosocial system, the clinician may call upon this system to cope with the family or individual crisis. Second, where an exceptionally well-developed and strong dysfunctional system exists, the clinician may aim to treat the psychosocial system as a dysfunctional unit. Third, where the psychosocial system is the primary system without a nuclear family constellation, the clinician may treat the functional psychosocial system identified by the nominal patient. Fourth, where a neurotic psychosocial system exists, it may be possible to repopulate the system with real people rather than dead or absent people, and to resolve the negativistic relations that do exist. Fifth, with a psychotic psychosocial system, it may be important for the clinician to open up the totally closed system and establish interpersonal relations with other social subsystems so that an effective psychosocial system can be established.

TOWARD A CLINICAL THEORY FOR SOCIAL SYSTEM THERAPY

The purpose of this section is to describe a theoretical approach to psychotherapy based on social system theory. This approach is neither psychological nor sociological. Rather, I view human behavior as the *product* of an interaction between individual psychology and the social field. Hence I use the term *psychosocial* to label the *system of behavior*.

I define therapy as a healing intervention on behalf of a *specific individual* who has identifiable dysfunctional behavior. This may be internal behavior (thoughts, feelings) or external behavior (words, actions). There are other healing interventions in the history of medicine that are quite properly conducted on the behalf of people in general, such as water fluoridation, vitamin enrichment of bread, public sanitation, etc. Such general system interventions, without a specific individual target, might be termed medical care, but not medical therapy.

In terms of mental health, I deem it important to distinguish levels of system intervention, some of which are therapy, others of which are care. Still other levels of system intervention that utilize mental health skills and knowledge are not properly subsumed under a sickness-health paradigm because different social sanctions and norms operate to regulate professional intervention. For example, organizational consultation is often provided by mental health consultants. The social sanction is not based on a "sick" organization that requires "healing." Rather, the mental health professional offers skills and knowledge from one professional arena that may be useful in another arena but under a nonmedical set of role norms.

There is a clear social sanction to define certain individual behavior as "sick" in terms of mental health parameters. There is also social sanction to "treat" the sick individual. Currently in the development of mental health concepts we have moved toward a more social view of human behavior. In so doing, we seek social sanction to define and treat a social unit comprised of more than one person.

We have gained social sanction to define and treat "sick" families as a social unit. At this point there is much conceptual confusion. On the one hand, critics maintain that only an individual can appropriately be defined as sick, and that a social unit cannot be labeled as sick. On the other hand, some family therapists assert that there are no sick individuals, only sick families; the individual psychopathology is defined as a reflection of the family. Thus if the family were well, the individual would be well.

For my part, I take neither position. The social purpose of defining a person of a social unit as sick is integral to the social sanction to treat that person or social unit. Thus we may label any social unit, family, neighborhood community, organization, city, or government as sick. But we do not have the social sanction to do so, nor do we have the social sanction for treatment intervention. We gain social sanction to define and treat to the extent we can demonstrate appropriate skills and knowledge that justify a social mandate to treat.

The professional mandate for treatment is rooted in the individual.

The farther we depart from the individual, the weaker the social mandate to define and intervene. Family therapy did not develop because of the discovery of sick families, but rather from the demonstration that the family was inextricably linked with the defined sick individual. We have demonstrated that intervention with the family produced healing of the individual. We have thus gained sanction to define the family social system as sick and engage in family treatment *as a system*.

Therefore, we can define an individual as sick, and we can define a family as sick. But we do not have a mandate to treat a sick family that has no identifiable sick individual. But let us go a step further. The *degree* of intimate relationship between the individual and a social unit is critical to the extension of a treatment mandate. For example, grandparents and cousins of a sick individual may be closely linked and properly involved in treatment. But if grandparents and cousins are not involved in the family life of the individual, they may properly disclaim involvement. The extreme end of this process is the sick worker in an office staff. Here it would usually be difficult to link the social unit of office staff behavior to the genesis and maintenance of individual sick behavior. Similarly, the office staff would probably disclaim involvement in the treatment of the individual. And surely we would have an impossible task to gain social sanction to define the office staff as sick and "treat" the office staff.

In this section, I am concerned with the extension of the social mandate to define and treat *social system units*. However, I wish to carefully differentiate the professional mandate for treatment intervention.

The inception of psychotherapy at the turn of the century was based on the germ theory of illness. There was one person who had one germ that produced one syndrome of illness. Treatment was provided by the medical specialist who administered technical procedures upon the patient. Thus psychotherapy, based on this model, was a technical procedure that one specialist performed upon one person. Psychotherapeutic methods have moved from the one-to-one dyad of psychoanalysis to multiperson, multirelationship modes of psychotherapy contingent upon the effective interaction of a social system of people.

It is apparent that a social system approach to therapy stands a far distance from psychotherapy as defined by the one-to-one situation. More importantly, the attempt to "fit" social system therapy techniques within the conceptual domain of individual psychotherapy is not only herculean but inappropriate. Rather, I suggest that we need to devise a new conceptual model of psychotherapy for social system intervention, appropriate to these techniques. I thus propose two models of psychotherapy: a "personal" model and a "system" model. I see these two models of psychotherapy as complementary, rather than competitive, for they have different treatment goals and methods.

Gardner Murphy has observed that from the time of Aristotle until late in the nineteenth century, psychology was the study of individual minds. Group interaction and interpersonal relations were problems for the historian, the moralist, the jurist, the political economist. Psychotherapy was born in an intellectual era in which perhaps only a one-to-one model of psychotherapy could have been built. However, a social psychology of human relationships built on the work of William McDougall, Cooley, Durkheim, Giddings, Ross, Tonnies, and especially George Herbert Mead began to stir an intellectual ferment that was to shake psychological thinking loose from its individualistic moorings.

In the 1920's social scientists began to study "natural groups" in society, based on the conviction that the solution to "social problems" could be facilitated by the study of social interaction and normal social groupings. This empirical research approach was translated into social-work practice with groups. But interestingly, the "social group work" method has remained defined as *not* psychotherapy. The empirical study of natural groups in the community also gave rise to social welfare and social action programs. Yet here also such intervention was not defined as psychotherapeutic. In both instances, because specific people were not identified as "sick," these types of intervention were not seen as having therapeutic potential.

Finally, in the 1930's Kurt Lewin formulated his now famous "field theory." In brief, field theory posits that each individual exists in an interpersonal field of relationships. Each person exerts an influence on every other person in that field. But in addition, each person exists at a particular place in that field, with a cumulative effect on him from the juxtaposition of all around him. Lewin uses the term "valence" to symbolize the positive and negative tugs and pulls that impinge like magnetic forces upon the individual.

Lewin proposed that the behavior of the individual is the product of two forces. One is the internal psychological structure of the person. The other is field characteristics.

One can change behavior in two ways. First, we can intervene in the internal psychological structure of the individual. This is the traditional model of "personal" psychotherapy. The second method consists of intervention with the social field, such that the individual exists in a different field. This is the model of "system" therapy.

The early development of multiperson therapeutic situations may be seen as an application of general principles of Lewinian field theory. Other extensions of field theory are exemplified in small-group sociology, social psychology, and role theory. Persons operate in a social field which to a significant extent determines behavior. Thus one can create a social field of therapeutic benefit to the emotionally disturbed person. Cody Marsh, pioneer in group therapy methods, coined a succinct motto of this theory: "by the crowd they have been broken; by the crowd they shall be healed."

However, this concept of social field is an impersonal concept. The destructive or beneficent effects of the social field are not dependent on the particular personalities or relationships of the individual persons that comprise the field—rather it is the sociological structure of the field that determines its impact. Cody Marsh was thus quite correct when he used the word "crowd" in his aphorism.

When, however, we shift the focus of clinical concern to families and persons linked together by their instrumental and affective relationships to each other, we observe a more complex and different sociodynamic. For here we have not only the effects of impersonal sociological group function, but also the effects of instrumental and affective linkages that exist between members.

Edward Jay (130), an anthropologist, attempts to differentiate between the *impersonal social field* and the *personal psychosocial network*. He suggests that in a social field: "There is no hierarchy, no nucleated denser focus of relationship or center. The only center would be the unit from which we are looking outward in a given arbitrary distance. Every unit is in this sense a center. The units of the field may be individuals, families, communities, or other social aggregates, but the field as such does not constitute a 'group' with corporate qualities and cohesiveness." In contrast, Jay defines a network as the totality of all the units *connected by a certain type of relationship*. A network has definite boundaries. The focus of study of such a psychosocial network, then, is on the nature and quality of these specific connecting relationships that set the particular pattern of the network. For example, a family is a social network characterized primarily by specific affective connections, whereas a factory work team is a social network characterized primarily by specific instrumental connections.

What we have observed over the past 30 years is a step-by-step recognition of the psychosocial network in which the patient is embedded; moving from parents and child to nuclear family, to extended family, and finally to a complex social network that may include nuclear family, various kin, friends who have "affective" links, and persons like ministers and bosses who have "instrumental" links.

The major conceptual shift so far as therapy is concerned revolves around the focus of therapeutic intervention. In the one-to-one, personal model, the assumption is made that psychotherapy will effect change in the individual that will enable him to behave differently in his social fields and social networks. In contrast, in the multiple-person system model, we assume that by tightening and loosening the affective and instrumental linkages that exist in the network, different options for behavior will be presented to the "patient" and consequently the patient will behave differently. Thus, the focus of psychotherapy in the system model is to change the interactional characteristics of the psychosocial network. This model explicitly assumes that human behavior is significantly determined by the characteristics of the social field or social network—hence the therapeutic emphasis lies here, rather than on changing the individual per se.

There are at least two major corollaries to this thesis. First, in the one-to-one, personal model, the definition of normality is essentially an *idealistic* one, i.e., the mature genital character, whereas in the system model the definition of normality is an *adaptive* one, i.e., capacity to operate effectively in the person's social field and network. Second, the personal model focuses on characterological change, whereas the system model focuses on behavioral change.

THE PERSONAL VERSUS SOCIAL MODEL

I shall now briefly outline some distinct differences between a personal and system model of psychotherapy. My aim is to illustrate that the two models do not compete, but rather are complementary models, for each is addressed to different psychotherapeutic goals.

The system model of psychotherapy is actually the oldest. It is the model of the shaman, the primitive healer, the folk healer. In primitive society if a member became "sick," this was matter for public concern, for a necessary worker was lost to the small society. Hence it was in the interest of everyone to see to it that the sick person was restored to function. There was little margin for functionless members of the community; everyone was needed to keep the small society functional. When a person became emotionally "ill," there was a generally accepted societal explanation for the cause of the illness. Further, everyone in the small society knew what healing procedures needed to be carried out. And everyone knew what the shaman would do in his healing rituals.

The goal of the healing was to restore the ill person to his usual mode of operation and function in the social system. There was no questioning of the values or patterns of function of the social system.

In other words, there was a value consensus between healer-patient-society. And there was a healing consensus between healer-patient-society. The healing procedures were a multiperson enterprise that involved healer-patient-society.

In contrast, the personal model of psychotherapy developed with quite a different rationale. The goal was not to help the patient return to function in his social system in the same old way. Rather, it was to help the patient to examine his social system, examine his pattern of function in his social system, and perhaps function in a different social system altogether.

Now the personal model could only come into existence in the face of several other social considerations. First, the person was not immediately required for the society to function, he could remain dysfunctional for extended periods of time. Second, the person had available to him a variety of value systems from which he could choose, i.e., he did not live in a one-value society. And third, the person had available alternative social systems into which he could move.

In the system model, privacy is antitherapeutic, for it is the public pressure, public response, and public support that enables the person to move rapidly back into his accustomed social function. In the personal model privacy is paramount, for it is the privacy that enables the person to achieve distance and perspective on his behavior in his social system. It is the privacy of the personal model that allows the patient to explore alternatives without public pressure, with public response, and without public support.

Thus we can see that if our psychotherapeutic goal is rapid return of a "sick" person to accustomed social function, then we may choose the system model to capitalize on the "public" that comprises the patient's social system. This is psychosocial system therapy. It is a public therapy. The difference between the primitive shaman and the psychosocial-system-model therapist is that the therapist may aim at changing some characteristics of the social system, not merely using the social system as does the primitive shaman.

If our psychotherapeutic goal is change of personality with the concomitant development of capacity to choose among alternative social systems, then the personal model of psychotherapy in the traditional psychoanalytic sense becomes the model of choice.

The advantage of having two models of psychotherapy is that the psychotherapist may be freed from the attempt to make very different types of therapeutic interventions fit into a model that is inappropriate (hence experiencing conflict over a variety of technical, social, and ethical issues). Further, the psychotherapist can clearly

Table 3
Two Complementary Models of Psychotherapy

	Personal Model	System Model
GPA:	To change personality structure	To reinforce adaptive personality structure
Patient relation to social system	May choose to change social systems	Seeks to return to social system
Therapist relation to social system	Is given social sanction to stand apart and question	Is given social sanction to help social system function better
Psychotherapy vis-a-vis the social system	Occurs at a distance	Occurs in ongoing system
Privacy of psychotherapy	Of paramount importance	Antitherapeutic
Members of psychotherapy	Therapist and patient	Therapist and social system
Focus of psychotherapy	Individual patient (patient directly)	Total social system (patient indirectly)
Role of psychotherapist	To catalyze capacity of patient to develop self-direction	To catalyze capacity of social system to function more effectively
Definition of patient	Self-defined, or deviant as defined by society	Secondary to definition of social system
Definition of therapist	Professionally defined role	Secondary to definition of responsible social system

take advantage of the strengths of either model, instead of compromising one model to achieve the goals of the other model.

The differences between the two models are charted in Table 3 for comparative purposes.

TOWARD A CLINICAL TYPOLOGY OF SOCIAL SYSTEMS TREATMENT

In this final section, I would like to tie together the several frames of reference developed in this paper into a clinical typology. In so doing, I wish to illustrate where we may logically place different types of clinical treatment strategies. Furthermore, I wish to delineate the matter of boundaries and contracts. Lieberman (131) has recently pointed out that people seek help from many systems in the community.

The major difference in where they seek help is not in the goals, but in their perception of how changes will take place and who will help them. Both Singer et al. (132) and Lieberman and Gardner (133) have pointed out that the boundaries between treatment and non-treatment methods and groups have been blurred. Thus the issue from a systems point of view is not what is or is not treatment, but rather a question of definition of system boundaries and system contracts. In a word, we must define the social role of the mental health professional vis-à-vis intervention in different types of social systems. These dimensions are shown in Table 4.

Since my premise is based on treatment intervention on behalf of the identified individual, I shall frame my typology in terms of the *subjective network* and the zones of intimacy and relatedness to the individual. We shall move from the most intimate zone of social system intervention to the most impersonal, extended zone of relations.

The Primary Family Unit—First-Zone Intervention

As you will recall, the first zone of relations usually consists of the nuclear family constellation. Family therapy would be the social system intervention here. The goal of family therapy is to achieve structural change in the family style of operation as a system (38). Variant methods may be used to enhance the learning and change process of the nuclear family. This would include married couples group therapy (3) and multiple family therapy (4–6). These latter methods try to enhance the therapeutic process through observation and interaction with similar social units. The professional is therapist of the social system.

The Intimate Psychosocial System— First-Second-Zone Interventions

Here we deal with the functional psychosocial system. Up to this point, the system has been usually defined by the "category" set, namely, who is related to the nuclear family by blood or marriage. The method is thus an extension of nuclear family therapy applied and modified to meet the needs of a modified kinship family structure. Minuchin et al. (36) and Boszormenyi-Nagy and Spark (39) represent therapists of the extended family system. Sager et al. (35) are transitional therapists who still conduct family psychotherapy with an extended family system, but that system may include such functional kin as neighbors, co-workers, community residents, etc.

Pattison (27, 28) approaches direct psychotherapy of the psychosocial kinship unit, which is formally composed of the egocentric-defined, personal network of the defined patient. In contrast to those above, who use a "category" set, Pattison uses a "personal" set to define the psychosocial kinship system.

Finally, there is the "network therapy" of Attneave (16), Speck (10, 31), Speck and Attneave (33), Ruevini (34), and Ruevini and Speck (30). They also use a "personal" set. However, they differ from Pattison in that they do not necessarily attempt to change the structural function of the psychosocial system as Pattison does. Rather, they define their work as mobilizing the system to respond effectively to the patient. Further, Attneave, Speck, and Ruevini do not limit their work to the intimate psychosocial network of first and second zones, but may work briefly with up to 100 people including third- and fourth-zone people.

The Temporary Psychosocial System— Quasi–First-Second-Zone Interventions

Here we deal with situations where there is no adequate psycho-social system or a very dysfunctional system that provides a healthy approximation of a social system. I have in mind the therapeutic community devised by Maxwell Jones (66) to treat sociopathic disorders, the therapeutic communities and Synanon for the treatment of drug addicts, and the hospital and day-care social rehabilitation programs for schizophrenics (134).

These social systems provide a temporary social system for those patients who need an intensive rehabilitative experience. The therapist here does not treat the patient, but directs the system so that it provides a healthy milieu for psychological stabilization. Thus he is the therapist of the system. Indeed this has been called "sociotherapy." We may also note that some people cannot return directly to community life, and may be provided an ongoing temporary psychosocial system, such as the half-way houses for alcoholics and the therapeutic lodges for schizophrenics (72, 135).

The Ecological System—Third-Fourth-Fifth-Zone Interventions

This social system is not a face-to-face interactional group, but rather a linkage of persons who provide a discrete set of services. That is, who is linked to a patient, or can be linked to a patient, in order to catalyze the provision of useful affective and instrumental support? The intent of this type of system intervention is to assemble an effective response network. Thus people in zones 3–5 may be

Table 4
Summary of Social-System Intervention Systems

	Personal System	Intimate Psychosocial System	Temporary Psychosocial System	Ecological System	Replacement System	Participation System
Personal Zone	1	1-2	1-2	1-5	3-4	4-5
Type of Network	Personal Set	Personal Set	Categorical Set	Action Set	Role-System Set	Field Set
Time Set	Ongoing	Ongoing	Temporary	Time-limited to action	Time-limited to life problem	Maybe limited or ongoing
Intimacy of Systems	Total	High	High in context	Limited to action	Limited to problem	Informed
Interaction of Subject with System	Total life	Frequent over total life	Total in context	Based on action	Partial and selective	Highly selective
Role of Professional	Therapist of system	Type A Therapist of system	System director	System coordinator	System collaborator	System cooperator

Clinician Examples	Family therapists Minuchin Sager	Type B Convener/ interviewer of system Type A Pattison Type B Speck Ruevini Attneave	Day-care Synanon Maxwell Jones	Auerswald Garrison Hansell Polak	Partial Groups A.A. Self-help groups Substitute Groups Big Brother-Big Sister Crisis groups	Social clubs Recreation groups Churches Service clubs
Named Clinical Intervention	Extended family therapy	Network therapy	Therapeutic communities	Screening Planning Community- linking	Therapeutic natural com- munity groups	Voluntary community associations

assembled in one place to organize and plan an effective response to the patient. Such a conference might include a psychotherapist, a probation officer, a school teacher, a pastor, neighbors, family, and relatives. The aim is to achieve communication and congruence of goals among all the people with whom the patient may have contact. As a result, the patient will be able to identify the "ecological niches" where each person, agency, service, resource is located. And then the patient will be able to utilize the resources provided through explicit linking of the patient with each person in each ecological niche in the community. Representative therapists of this method include Auerswald (17, 18), Callan et al. (19), Hansell (76, 77), Hansell et al. (78), Garrison (22), Nadler (136), and Polak (29). It is here that paraprofessionals may be used as ombudsman to assist the patient to identify and utilize the people in this community ecological network of resources (137–140). The professional here is a "system coordinator." This system is both personal and impersonal in its network connections.

The Kin-Replacement System—Third-Fourth-Zone Interventions

In this instance we look at social systems in which the patient has partial participation on an intimate basis. Here we face the problem of the patient who lacks an available number of people to recruit into his social network, to provide affective and instrumental care. Hence part-time replacements are necessary. There are two subtypes.

The ongoing partial replacement system

This kind of system is best exemplified in self-help groups. The self-help group does not become involved with the totality of the person's life, but does provide socialization, support, guidance, and assistance around specific life problems, such as alcoholism, child abuse, divorce. The self-help group does not involve the totality of possible life actions as does the intimate psychosocial system, but remains identified with the problem behavior (141, 142).

The time-limited substitution system

In this type of system, the person is offered a more total relationship to meet an intercurrent stress or crisis, but the system is available only on a time-limited basis to substitute for the lack of a personal social network. Examples include Big Brothers and Big Sisters programs, widow-to-widow programs, and crisis-intervention groups (85, 88, 143, 144).

In both subtypes of kin replacement, the professional plays the role of "system collaborator," in which he aids the patient to become involved in such a replacement system.

The Associational System—Fourth- and Fifth-Zone Interventions

Here I refer to social systems that offer both instrumental and affective support on a less intimate and less global basis. The social systems here are voluntary associations. Examples would include ad hoc systems like tavern groups, street-corner gangs, and school cliques, and organized systems like church groups, Great Books clubs, social clubs, service organizations, and recreational associations (145–150).

Although such voluntary social systems have other social aims and functions aside from psychological support per se, they also provide a rich social matrix for less intimate but nonetheless important human relationships (151). The data from social anthropology suggest that participation in voluntary associations is in part an adaptive attempt to construct viable kinship systems. Thus these systems of voluntary association became a replenishment resource. The professional relates to these systems as a "system cooperator."

To summarize: Each of the six types of social systems bears a different relationship to the target individual. As we move from the most to the least intimate system, the embeddedness and connectedness of the person in that system decreases. Yet each system may be of clinical relevance to the coping capacity of the individual at a given point.

In similar fashion, the mental health professional has a different relationship with each of the six types. His strongest mandate for intervention is with the most intimate system, and his mandate decreases as the systems become more impersonal and distant from the target patient. The role of the professional is, respectively, system treatment agent, system treatment director, system coordinator, system collaborator, and finally, system cooperator.

I do not wish to define each of these systems as "treatment systems." For each system is not a treatment system, nor does the professional have a mandate to treat each system. And of course, most importantly, the issue is not treatment of each system, but rather how the professional can functionally relate to each system in order to achieve system benefits for the patient. I have thus tried to illustrate how the professional plays different roles vis-à-vis the system so that the patient can appropriately participate in and utilize each social system.

SUMMARY

This chapter has set forth the rationale for clinical interventions in the social system of community life. Theoretical and empirical data have been gathered to formulate a middle-range set of constructs and theory that link the individual to social process. Finally, a formal typology is presented to organize clinical interventions in accord with the theory of social systems.

REFERENCES

1. Speigel, J.P. The family: The channel of primary care. *Hosp. Commun. Psychiat.*, 25: 785, 1974.
2. Bell, N.W. Extended family relations of disturbed and well families. *Fam. Process*, 1: 175–193, 1962.
3. Gottlieb, A., and Pattison, E.M. Married couples group psychotherapy. *Arch. Gen. Psychiat.*, 14: 143–152, 1966.
4. Barcai, A. An adventure in multiple family therapy. *Fam. Process*, 6: 185–192, 1967.
5. Blinder, M.G. Colman, A.D., Curry, A.E., and Kessler, D.R. MCFT: Simultaneous treatment of severe families. *Amer. J. Psychother.*, 19: 559–569, 1965.
6. Curry, A.E. Therapeutic management of multiple family groups. *Internat. J. Group Psychother.*, 15: 90*96, 1965.
7. Laquer, H.P. General systems theory and multiple family therapy. In: *Current Psychiatric Therapies*, Vol. 8, ed. J.H. Masserman. New York: Grune and Stratton, 1968.
8. Pattison, E.M. Treatment of alcoholic families with nurse home visits. *Fam. Process*, 4: 75–94, 1965.
9. Perry, S.E. Home treatment and the social system of psychiatry. *Psychiatry*, 26: 54–64, 1963.
10. Speck, R.V., Family therapy in the home. *J. Marr. Fam. Living*, 26: 72–76, 1964.
11. Hansen, C.C. An extended home visit with conjoint family therapy. *Fam. Process*, 7: 67–87, 1968.
12. Lidz, T., Fleck, S., and Cornelison, A.R. The limitations of extrafamilial socialization. In: *Schizophrenia and the Family*. New York: International Universities Press, 1965, Chap. 18.
13. Mac Gregor, R., Ritchie, A.M., Serrano A.C., and Schuster, F.P. *Multiple Impact Therapy with Families*. New York: McGraw-Hill 1964.
14. Weiner, L., Becker, A., and Friedman T. *Home Treatment*. Pittsburgh: University of Pittsburgh Press, 1967.
15. Alissi, A.S. Social work with families in group-service agencies: An overview. *Fam. Coordinator*, 18: 391–401, 1969.

16. Attneave, C.L. Therapy in tribal settings and urban network intervention. *Fam. Process*, 8: 192–210, 1969.
17. Auerswald, E.H. Interdisciplinary versus ecological approach. *Fam. Process*, 7: 202–215, 1968.
18. Auerswald, E. Families, change and the ecological perspective. In: *Family Therapy Textbook*, ed. A. Ferber, M. Mendelsohn, and A. Napier. Boston: Houghton Mifflin, 1972.
19. Callan, D., Garrison, J., and Zerger, F. Working with the families and social networks of drug abusers. *J. Psychedel. Drugs*, 7: 19–26, 1975.
20. Finlay, D.G. Effect of role network pressures on an alcoholic's approach to treatment. *Soc. Work*, 11: 71–77, 1966.
21. Friedman, P.H. Family system and ecological approach to youthful drug abuse. *Fam. Therapy*, 7: 63–78, 1974.
22. Garrison, J. Network techniques: Case studies in the screening–linking–planning conference method. *Fam. Process*, 13: 337–353, 1974.
23. Hoffman, L., and Long, L. A system dilemma. *Fam. Process*, 8: 211–234, 1969.
24. Landes, J., and Winter, W. A new strategy for treating disintegrated families. *Fam. Process*, 5: 1–20, 1966.
25. Laskin, E. Breaking down the walls. *Fam. Process*, 7: 118–125, 1968.
26. Mannino, E.V., and Shore, M.F. Ecologically oriented family interaction. *Fam. Process*, 11: 499–505, 1972.
27. Pattison, E.M. Social system psychotherapy. *Amer. J. Psychother.*, 17: 396–409, 1973.
28. Pattison, E.M. Group treatment methods suitable for family practice. *Internat. Pub. Health Rev.*, 2: 247–265, 1973.
29. Polak, P. Social systems intervention. *Arch. Gen. Psychiat.*, 25: 110–117, 1971.
30. Rueveni, U., and Speck, R.V. Using encounter group techniques in the treatment of the social network of the schizophrenic. *Internat. J. Group Psychother.*, 19: 495–500, 1971.
31. Speck, R.V. Psychotherapy of the social network of a schizophrenic family. *Fam. Proces*, 6: 208–214, 1967.
32. Speck, R.V., and Rueveni, U. Network therapy—a developing concept. *Fam. Process*, 8: 182–191, 1969.
33. Speck, R., and Attneave, C. *Family Networks*. New York: Panthenon, 1973.
34. Ruevini, U. Network intervention with a family crisis. *Fam. Process*, 14: 193–204, 1975.
35. Sager, C.J., Brayboy, T.L., and Waxenberg, B.R. *Black Ghetto Family in Therapy*. New York: Grove Press, 1970.
36. Minuchin, S., Montalvo, B., Guerney, B.C., Rosman, B.L., and Schumer, F. *Families of the Slums*. New York: Basic Books 1967.
37. Minuchin, S. The use of an ecological framework with treatment of the child. In: *The Child and His Family*, ed. E. Anthony and C. Koupernik. New York: Wiley-Interscience, 1970.

38. Boszormenyi-Nagy, I., and Framo, J.L. (eds.) A theory of relationships: Experiences and transactions. In: *Intensive Family Therapy*. New York: Hoeber, 1965, Chap. 2.
39. Boszormenyi-Nagy, I., and Spark, G.M. *Invisible Loyalties*. Hagerstown, Md.: Harper and Row, 1973.
40. Pattison, E.M. Psychosocial system therapy. In: *The Changing Mental Health Scene*. New York: Spectrum Press, 1976.
41. Pattison, E.M., De Francisco, D., Wood, P., Frazier, H., and Crowder, J. A psychosocial kinship model for family therapy. *Amer. J. Psychiat.*, 132: 1246–1251, 1975.
42. Adams, B.N. Isolation, function, and beyond: American kinship in the 1970's. *J. Marr. Fam. Living*, 32: 575–597, 1970.
43. Faris, R. Interaction of generations and family stability. *Amer. Sociol. Rev.*, 12: 159–164, 1947.
44. Sussman, M.B. The isolated nuclear family: Fact or fiction. *Soc. Prob.*, 6: 333–340, 1959.
45. Parsons, T. The kinship system of the contemporary United States. *Amer. Anthropol.* 45: 22–38, 1943.
46. Komarovsky, M. The voluntry associations of urban dwellers. *Amer. Sociol. Rev.*, 11: 686–698, 1946.
47. Dotson, F. Patterns of voluntary associations among urban working-class families. *Amer. Sociol. Rev.*, 16: 687–693, 1951.
48. Adams, B.N. Interaction theory and the social network. *Sociometry*, 30: 64–78, 1967.
49. Bott, E. Urban families: Conjugal roles and social network. *Hum. Relat.*, 8: 345–384, 1955.
50. Bott, E. *Family and Social Network*. London: Tavistock, 1957.
51. Gans, H.J. *The Urban Villagers*. New York: Free Press, 1962.
52. Gans, H.J. *The Levittowners*. New York: Pantheon, 1967.
53. Cohen, A.K., Hodges, H.M., Jr. Characteristics of the lower-blue-collar class. *Soc. Prob.*, 10: 303–334, 1963.
54. Farber, B. *Kinship and Family Organization*. New York: Wiley, 1966.
55. Hader, M. The importance of grandparents in family life. *Fam. Process*, 4: 228–240, 1965.
56. Hill, R. *Family Development in Three Generations*. Cambridge, Mass.: Schenkman, 1970.
57. Litwak, E. Extended kin relations in an industrial democratic society. In: *Social Structure and the Family: Generational Relations*, ed. E. Shanas, and G.F. Streib. Englewood Cliffs, N.J.: Prentice-Hall, 1965.
58. Reiss, P.J. The extended family system: Correlates of and attitudes on frequency of interaction. *J. Marr. Fam. Living*, 24: 333–339, 1962.
59. Shanas, E., and Streib, G.F. (eds.). Social structure and the family. In: *Generational Relations*. Englewood Cliffs, N.J.: Prentice-Hall, 1965.
60. Sussman, M.B., and Burchinal, L.G. Kinship family network: Unheralded structure in current conceptualization of family functioning. *J. Marr. Fam. Living*, 24: 231–240, 1962.

61. Sussman, M.B., and Burchinal, L. Parental aid to married children: Implications for family planning. *J. Marr. Fam. Living*, 24: 320–332, 1962.
62. Young, M., and Willmott, P. *Family and Kinship in East London*. London: Routledge and Kegan Paul, 1957.
63. Pattison, E.M. Group psychotherapy and group methods in community mental health. *Internat. J. Group Psychother.*, 21: 214–225, 1971.
64. Pattison, E.M. Systems pastoral care. *J. Pastoral Care*, 26: 2–14, 1972.
65. Caplan, G. *Support Systems and Community Mental Health*. New York: Behavioral Publications, 1974.
66. Jones, M. *Beyond the Therapeutic Community: Social Learning and Social Psychiatry*. New Haven: Yale University Press, 1968.
67. Klein, D.F. *Group Dynamics and Community Mental Health*. New York: Wiley, 1968.
68. Peck, H.B. The small group: Core of the community mental health center. *Commun. Ment. Health J.*, 4: 191–200, 1968.
69. Peck, H.B., and Kaplan, S. Crisis theory and therapeutic change in small groups: Some implications for community mental health programs. *Internat. J. Group Psychother.*, 16: 135–149, 1966.
70. Peck, H.B., Kaplan, S., and Roman, M. Prevention, treatment, and social action: A strategy of intervention in a disadvantaged urban area. *Amer. J. Orthopsychiat.*, 36: 57–69, 1966.
71. Blackman, S., and Goldstein, K.M. Some aspects of a theory of community mental health. *Commun. Ment. Health J.*, 4: 85–90, 1968.
72. Fairweather, G.W., Danders, D.H., Cressler, D.L., and Maynard, H. *Community Life for the Mentally Ill*. Chicago: Aldine, 1969.
73. Festinger, L., Schachter, S., and Back, K.W. *Social Pressures in Informal Groups*. New York: Harper, 1950.
74. Homan, G.C. *The Human Group*. New York: Harcourt Brace and World, 1950.
75. Phillips, M. *Small Social Groups in England*. London: Methuen, 1965.
76. Hansell, N. Patient predicament and clinical service: A system. *Arch. Gen. Psychiat.*, 14: 204–210, 1967.
77. Hansell, N. Casualty management method. *Arch. Gen. Psychiat.* 19: 281–289, 1968.
78. Hansell, N., Wodarczky, M., and Handlon-Lathrop, B. Decision counseling method: Expanding coping at crisis in transit. *Arch. Gen. Psychiat.*, 22: 462–467, 1970.
79. Collins, A.H. Natural delivery systems: Accessible sources of power for mental health. *Amer. J. Orthopsychiat.*, 43: 46–52, 1973.
80. Curtis, W.R. Community human service networks. *Psychiat. Ann.*, 3: 23–40, 1973.
81. Dillon, J. Community mental health in a rural region. In: *American Handbook of Psychiatry*, 2nd ed., Vol. 2, ed. G. Caplan. New York: Basic Books, 1974.
82. Woodbury, M.A. The Healing Team and Schizophrenia. In: *Psychiatric Hospital to Community Centered Intervention*. Springfield, Ill.: Thomas,

1969.
83. Woodbury, M.A., and Woodbury, M.M. Community-centered psychiatric intervention: A pilot project in the 13th arrondissement, Paris. *Amer. J. Psychiat.*, 126: 619–625, 1969.

84. Pringle, B.M. Family clusters as a means of reducing isolation among urbanites. *Fam. Coord.*, 23: 175–180, 1974.

85. Silverman, P. The widow as a caregiver in a program of preventive intervention with other widows. *Ment. Hygiene*, 54: 540–547, 1970.

86. Siporin, M. Social treatment: A new-old helping method. *Soc. Work*, 15: 13–25, 1970.

87. Sirporin, M. Situation assessment and intervention. *Soc. Casework*, 6: 91–109, 1972.

88. Zusman, J. "No-therapy": A method of helping persons with problems. *Commun. Ment. Health J.*, 5: 482–486, 1969.

89. Pattison, E.M. The role of adjunctive therapies in community mental health center programs. *Ther. Rec. J.*, 3: 16–25, 1969.

90. Doyle, E.C. Emerging community profiles. *J. Commun. Psychol.*, 3: 103–161, 1975.

91. Doyle, E.C., Brown, A.A. Community transaction analysis as a community-oriented research tool. *J. Commun. Psychol.*, 3: 358–364, 1975.

92. Gambrill, E.D. Role of behavior modification in community mental health. *Commun. Ment. Health J.*, 11: 307–315, 1975.

93. Weinstein, M., and Frankel, M. Ecological and psychological approaches to community psychology *.J. Commun. Psychol.*, 2: 43–52, 1974.

94. Baer, D., and Wolf, M. The entry into natural communities of reinforcement. In: *Control of Human Behavior*, Vol. 2, ed. R. Ulrich, T. Stachnick, and J. Mabry. Glenview, Ill.: Scott Foresman, 1970.

95. Boissevain, J. *Friends of Friends: Networks, Manipulators, and Coalitions.* New York: St. Martin's Press, 1974.

96. Boissevain, J., and Mitchell, J.C. (eds.). *Network Analysis: Studies in Human Interaction.* The Hague: Mouton, 1973.

97. Mitchell, J.C. (ed.). *Social Networks in Urban Situations.* Manchester, Eng.: Manchester University Press, 1969.

98. Whitten. N.E., Jr., and Wolfe, A.W. Network analysis. In: *The Handbook of Social and Cultural Anthropology*, ed. J. Honigmann. Chicago: Rand McNally, 1975.

99. Aldous, J. Intergenerational visiting patterns: Variations in boundary maintenance as an explanation. *Fam. Process*, 6: 235–251, 1967.

100. Bell, W., and Boat, M.D., Urban neighborhoods and informal social relations. *Amer. J. Sociol.*, 62: 391–398, 1957.

101. Bock, E.W., Iutaka, S., and Berardo, F.M. The maintenance of the extended family in urban areas of Argentina, Brazil, and Chile. *J. Comp. Fam. Stud.*, 6: 31–45, 1975.

102. Hsu, F.L.K. (ed.). *Kinship and Culture.* Chicago: Aldine, 1971.

103. Litwak, E., and Szelenyi, I. Primary group structures and their functions: Kin, neighbors, and friends. *Am. Sociol. Rev.*, 34: 465–481, 1969.

104. Sweetser, D. Mother-daughter ties between generations in industrial societies. *Fam. Process,* 3: 332–343, 1964.

105. Vatuk, S. *Kinship and Urbanization: White Collar Migrants in North India.* Berkeley: University of California Press, 1972.

106. Boswell, D.M. Personal crises and mobilization of social network. In: *Social Networks in Urban Situations,* ed. J.C. Mitchell. Manchester, Eng.: Manchester University Press, 1969.

107. Feldman, F., and Scherz, F. *Family Social Welfare.* New York: Atherton, 1967.

108. Litwak, E. The use of extended family groups in the achievement of social goals: Some policy implications. *Soc. Prob.,* 7: 177–187, 1959-1960.

109. Muir, D.E., and Weinstein, E.A. The social debt: An investigation of lower-class and middle-class norms of social obigation. *Amer. Sociol. Rev.,* 27: 532–539, 1962.

110. Young, M. The role of the extended family in disaster. *Hum. Relat.,* 7: 383–391, 1954.

111. Young, M. The extended family welfare association. *Soc. Work,* 13: 145–150, 1956.

112. Croog, S.H., Lipson, A., and Levine, S. Help patterns in severe illness: The roles of kin network, non-family resources, and institutions. *J. Marr. Fam. Living,* 34: 32–41, 1972.

113. McKinlay, J.B. Social networks, lay consultation, and help-seeking behavior. *Soc. Forces,* 51: 275–292, 1973.

114. Lebowitz, B.D., Fried, J., and Madaris, C. Sources of assistance in an urban ethnic community. *Hum. Org.,* 32: 267–271, 1973.

115. Salloway, J.C., and Dillon, P.B. A comparison of family network and friend network in health care utilization. *J. Comp. Fam. Stud.,* 4: 131–142, 1973.

116. Kammeyer, K.C.W., and Bolton, C.K. Community and family factors related to the use of a family service agency. *J. Marr. Fam. Living,* 30: 488–498, 1968.

117. Hammer, M. Influence of small social network as factors on mental hospital admission. *Hum. Org.,* 22: 243–251, 1963.

118. Brim, J.A. Social network correlates of avowed happiness. *J. Nerv. Ment. Dis.,* 158: 432–439, 1974.

119. Kleiner, R.J., and Parker, S. Network participation and psychosocial impairment in an urban environment. NIMH Grant MH 19897, Final Report, 1974.

120. Giavannoni, J.M., and Billingsley, A. Child neglect among the poor. *Child Welfare,* 69: 196–204, 1970.

121. Jackson, D.D. The individual and the larger contexts. *Fam. Process,* 6: 139–147, 1967.

122. Leichter, H.J., and Mitchell, W.E. *Kinship and Casework* New York: Russel Sage Foundation, 1967.

123. Mendell, D., and Fisher, S. An approach to neurotic behavior in terms

of a three generation family model. *J. Nerv. Ment. Dis.*, 123: 171–180, 1956.

124. Mendell, D., and Fisher, S. A multi-generational approach to treatment of psychopathology. *J. Nerv. Ment. Dis.*, 126: 523–529, 1958.

125. Mendell, D., Cleveland, S.E., and Fisher, S. A five-generation family theme. *Fam. Process*, 7: 126–132, 1968.

126. Ferraro, G.P. Some methodological observations on the study of urban kinship. *J. Comp. Fam. Stud.*, 5: 117–124, 1974.

127. Peterson, K.K. Kin network research: A plea for comparability. *J. Marr. Fam. Living*, 31: 271–280, 1969.

128. Yorburg, B. The nuclear and extended family in disaster. *Hum. Relat.*, 7: 383–391, 1975.

129. Killworth, P., and Bernard, H.R. Catij: A new sociometric and its application to a prison living unit. *Hum. Org.*, 33: 335–350, 1974.

130. Jay, E.J. The concepts of 'field' and 'network' in anthropological research. *Man*, 64: 137–139, 1964.

131. Lieberman, M.A. Some limits to research on T groups. *J. Appl. Behav. Sci.*, 11: 241–249, 1975.

132. Singer, D.L., Astrachan, B.M., Gould, L.J., and Klein, E.B. Boundary management in psychological work with groups. *J. Appl. Behav. Sci.*, 11: 137–177, 1975.

133. Lieberman, M.A., and Gardner, J. Institutional alternative to psychotherapy: A study of growth center users. *Arch. Gen. Psychiat.*, 33: 157–162, 1976.

134. Astrachan, B.M., Flynn, H.H., Geller, J.D., and Harvey, H.D. Systems approach to day hospitalization. *Arch. Gen. Psychiat.*, 22: 550–559, 1970.

135. Raush, H.L., and Raush, C.L. *The Halfway House Movement*. New York: Appleton-Century-Crofts, 1968.

136. Nadler, E. Social approaches to community mental health via intake or central receptive services. *Commun. Ment. Health J.*, 9: 361–367, 1973.

137. Cohen, R. The collaborative coprofessional: Developing a new mental health role. *Hosp. Comm. Psychiat.*, 24: 242–246, 1973.

138. Griffith, C., and Libo, L. *Mental Health Consultants: Agents of Community Change*. San Francisco: Jossey-Bass, 1968.

139. Torrey, E.F. The case for the indigenous therapist. *Arch. Gen. Psychiat.*, 20: 365–373, 1969.

140. Umbarger, C. The paraprofessional and family therapy. *Fam. Process*, 11: 147–162, 1972.

141. Ablon, J. Al-anon family groups. *Amer. J. Psychother.*, 19: 30–45, 1974.

142. Ryback, R.S. Schizophrenics anonymous: A treatment adjunct. *Psychiat. Med.* 2: 247–253, 1971.

143. Indin, B.M. The crisic club: A group experience for suicidal patients. *Ment. Hygiene*, 50: 280–290, 1966.

144. Strickler. M., and Allgeyer, J. The crisis group. A new application of crisis

theory. *Soc. Work*, 12: 28–32, 1969.

145. Alexander, W.B. The development of a therapeutic social club. *Hosp. Commun. Psychiat.*, 21: 230–233, 1970.

146. Brodsky, I. The role and function of the community recreation center in programs of socio-medical rehabilitation. *Brit. J. Soc. Psychiat.* 1: 189–199, 1967.

147. Dumont, M. Tavern culture: The sustenance of homeless men. *Amer. J. Orthopsychiat.*, 37: 938–945, 1967.

148. Goodenough, D. Self-study groups: Hope for the troubled normal. *Commun. Ment. Health J.*, 1: 184–187, 1965.

149. Merrill, T. *Social Clubs for the Aging.* Springfield, Ill.: Thomas, 1971.

150. Thompson, E.M. Therapeutic social clubs for chronic and disturbed patients. *Internat. J. Soc. Psychiat.*, 1: 37–41, 1956.

151. Smith, C., and Freedman, A. *Voluntary Associations*: *Perspectives on the Literature*. Cambridge, Mass.: Harvard University Press, 1972.

18

The Future of Cultural Psychiatry

JOHN J. SCHWAB
MARY E. SCHWAB

Although the term "cultural psychiatry" is not in common use, scholarly interest in culture and mental illness can be traced to the early decades of the nineteenth century when both psychiatry and anthropology emerged as disciplines. We think that concern for the future of cultural psychiatry requires an appreciation of the historical developments that led to a confluence of interest for workers in these fields. We shall therefore look first at some early studies in psychiatric epidemiology which were stimulated by turbulent changes in the sociopolitical climate, and include some rough transcultural comparisons. Then, taking into account the many theoretical advances in both anthropology and psychiatry during this century, we shall discuss some current views on cultural psychiatry and a few timely issues for research, present and future.

At the end of the eighteenth century, tumultuous sociopolitical events—industrialization, urbanization, the American and French Revolutions, and the flowering of sentiments espousing humanitarianism and the dignity of man—prompted studies to determine whether mental illness was increasing and to assess possible cultural influences on its frequency. Pioneers in psychiatric epidemiology, such as George Man Burrows, Andrew Halliday, and Jean Etienne Esquirol, gathered data on the number of mentally ill in various nations to pursue their inquiries into the nature of insanity and to evaluate the impact of the economic and political commotions of the times on mental health and illness in different countries.

In 1820, Burrows (1) concluded that insanity was not increasing in England and Wales although heightened interest in the ˙subject, produced by the tragic mental illness of George III and the crop failures, accounted for fluctuations in the number of admissions to mental hospitals in certain years. His study of case registers and hospital superintendents' reports indicated that the prevalence of mental illness probably was lower in Scotland than in England and Wales because of the "moral and intellectual character of the Scotch." He thought that the prevalence in Ireland was very high because of widespread deprivation and alcoholism.

In 1828, Andrew Halliday (2) presented *A General View of the Present State of Lunatics and Lunatic Asylums in Great Britain and Ireland, and in Some Other Kingdoms.* He believed that mental illness was rare in "the savage tribes" in Africa, the slaves in West Indies, and the "contented peasantry of the Welsh Mountains, the Western Hebrides, and the Wilds of Ireland" (p. 80). In contrast, mental illness was a serious, not uncommon malady in the civilized nations of Western Europe because of overexertion of the mind or bodily powers with consequent "derangement of the vital functions, that re-act upon the brain, and damage its operations." Thus, "cultural psychiatry" dawned with the belief that mental illness was a byproduct of civilization, a viewpoint which had been expressed by the ancients—Democritus in the fifth century B.C. and Lucretius four centuries later.

Esquirol (3), in the 1830's, along with Burrows and Halliday, thought that mental illness was caused by both hereditary and moral factors. In his studies of mental illness over four decades in France, he attempted to answer the question: Has insanity become more common since the French Revolution? He concluded that the observed increase was more apparent than real, attributable to improvements in facilities. But he added a disclaimer: possibly insanity was increasing during the 1820's and 1830's because of a greater laxity in moral standards. He stated:

There is no more domestic affection, nor respect, nor love, nor authority, nor reciprocal dependencies. Each lives for himself;

no one forming those wise combinations, which connect the present, with coming generations.... When we add to these causes the manner of life of the women in France ... together with the misery and privations of the lower classes, we shall no longer be astonished at the disorder of public and private morals, nor any longer have a right to complain, if nervous disorders, and particularly insanity, multiply in France (p. 350).

These are familiar notes in our contemporary society where dissent, drugs, and disease are attributed to permissiveness. And Esquirol's reflections, one and a half centuries ago, before the concept of culture had been elaborated, point out that man's cultural legacy—sentiments, customs, morals, and laws—is transmitted to subsequent generations and thereby influences their health.

The word "Kultur" (4) appeared first in German in 1793 about the same time that the towering intellect of the age, Immanuel Kant, designated "anthropology" as the scientific study of man, including his psychology. In 1871, the father of modern anthropology, Edward Tylor, established the word "culture," in its current technical sense, in English. Tylor (quoted in 4) defined culture as "... that complex whole which includes knowledge, belief, art, law, morals, custom, and any other capabilities and habits acquired by man as a member of society" (p. 81).

About the same time, Daniel Hack Tuke (5) reviewed the history of mental illness in prehistoric times, and among the Jews, Egyptians, Greeks, and Romans. He believed that even prehistoric and ancient societies were "no strangers to the inroads of mental disease" (p. 8). After gathering reports from missionaries and explorers, he concluded that mental illness was probably much rarer in primitive and uncivilized groups than in societies that attained highly developed cultures. However, in his remarkable volume, Tuke did not romanticize "the noble savage," extolled by Rousseau as enjoying the earth's "fruits and flowers without toil or worry" (p. 10). Instead, he quoted Voltaire's sarcastic retort to Rousseau: "Almost you persuade me to go on all fours" (p. 10).

Tuke believed that among the Egyptians, Greeks, and Romans the frequency of mental illness increased with the maturation of the society, particularly during its decadent period. But, insightfully, he pointed out that the insane were probably much fewer in number in ancient times than in the nineteenth century because life was probably more difficult in the past—those less able to adapt and those with feeble constitutions perished in infancy or childhood, or certain customs had limited the propagation of the mentally ill. In Palestine, for example, sons affected with moral insanity, manifested by disobedience to their parents or violation of the group's laws, were stoned to death. Homicidal men killed and were killed in the wars of Greece and Rome; and infanticide was a common practice used to stamp out cases of mental deficiency or derangement.

Tuke thought that insanity was increasing in Britain in the middle of the nineteenth century because of alcoholism, malnutrition, and other types of deprivation in the lower classes, and because of the corruption of morals, the use of stimulants, and the stresses of modern life in the upper classes. He believed that the complexity of modern life threatened to exceed the capacity of man's nervous system for adaptation. Yet he did not indict civilization per se, but its abuses, as the cause of increasing insanity. He said that civilization "... is simply the penalty which superior organisms have to pay for their greater sensitiveness and susceptibility. Civilisation involves risks because it entails a higher form of mental life, and our highest wisdom consists in thankfully accepting this boon and escaping one of these risks by the prevention of insanity" (p. 9).

Tuke's views were courageous. We should recall that he was writing at a time when Social Darwinism was flowering. His views were idiosyncratic, if not treasonous, in the complacent, self-righteous Victorian society of the 1870's which believed in progress and took pride in its assumed moral and industrial supremacy.

During the next 50 years, when modern psychiatry developed under the influence of Kraepelin, Freud, and Bleuler, psychiatrists and social scientists described some of the exotic and culture-bound syndromes. Freud conceptualized neurosis as a result of the struggle between the individual's instinctual drives and civilization's repressive processes and theorized about the development of the mental apparatus. The psychoanalytic model specified links between interpersonal and intrapsychic events and the mechanisms responsible for pathological outcomes. Anthropologists, traditionally concerned with the study of primitive cultures, were faced with the provocative question of whether this model applied for groups with social structures and interpersonal behavior codes vastly different from those in Western society.

Géza Róheim (6), a student of Freud, was one of the first anthropologists to try to determine the applicability of the psychoanalytic model in primitive groups. He found that the classical neuroses were rare in the Australian tribes he studied and conjectured that this was a result of the weaker intensity of repression in primitive races than in European societies. He believed in an ontogenetic view of culture and, in accord with Freud's philosophical speculations, analogized between the infant's psyche and the primitive tribe's cultural processes. He thought that continued comparative studies of groups in various stages of cultural development would show how the mind of modern man had evolved. Moreover, he believed that psychoanalytic anthropology would become a new science and that eventually the mind of the group, analogous to the mind of man, could be analyzed, hopefully with therapeutic results.

In contrast, Malinowski's (7) classic study of the Trobriand Islanders helped establish the school of functional anthropology. He and others found that child-rearing practices in various cultures differed considerably and that the classic Oedipus complex was not a universal phenomenon, but that personality disorders and deviations could be found in all societies.

Both psychiatrists and anthropologists now agree that mental illnesses exist in all cultures. For example, in discussing "The Future of Psychiatry," Leon Eisenberg (8) asserts that one of the strongest proofs against the "myth of mental illness" thesis is that, although explanations of the cause and nature of mental illness differ from culture to culture, all cultures "... recognize and label mental disorders." Anthony F. C. Wallace (9) states flatly that: "There are no human societies in which mental disorders, of one sort or another, never occur" (p. 367). And, after studying the Hutterites, Eaton and Weil (10) mention wistfully that there is no "mental health utopia."

During the last few decades, with contributions from archeology and social and biological anthropology, "the concept of culture" has been elaborated. In simple terms, Clyde Kluckhohn (11) states that culture is: (1) man's social legacy; (2) the part of the environment created by man; (3) a design for living; (4) the channel for biological processes; (5) a way of thinking, feeling, and behaving; (6) a group's distinctive ways of living; and (7) a regulator of our lives. Moreover, he maintains that cultures both produce needs and provide means for fulfilling them and also supply "a set of blueprints for human relations."

In their comprehensive work, *Culture: A Critical Review of Concepts and Definitions*, Kroeber and Kluckhohn (4) formulate culture as the "... patterns, explicit and implicit, of and for behavior acquired and transmitted by symbols, constituting the distinctive achievement of human groups, including their embodiments in artifacts; the essential core of culture consists of traditional ideas and especially their attached values; culture systems may, on the one hand, be considered as products of action, on the other as conditioning elements of further action" (p. 357).

Thus, we can see that the concept of culture is fundamental to our understanding of mental illness because man is a biosocial organism not only molded by his interactions with others and influenced by customs and the objects of his material culture, but also endowed with a cultural legacy. Moreover, the individual's biological, social, and spiritual needs and the means by which they are gratified, frustrated, or sublimated—the conflicts intrinsic to mental illness—are culturally as well as biologically determined. Any view of a mentally ill person that does not place him in a cultural perspective is bound to be myopic.

Kluckhohn states that cultures supply "blueprints for human relations"; these blueprints encompass pathological as well as healthy patterns. Just as the blueprints differ and change, the manifestations of mental disorder vary among such wide-ranging groups as Eskimos with piblokto, Southeastern Asiatics with amok, or Algonkian hunters with windigo psychosis. And they vary even among those in close proximity, as among ethnic groups in the United States. Wallace (12) notes: "Most such 'ethnic psychoses,' which reflect in their behavior the specific cultural content of the victim's society, are simply local varieties of a common disease process to which human beings are vulnerable. In this light, then, all mental disorders must be considered to reflect, in symptomatic content, the victim's past and present cultural environment" (pp. 218–219). Thus, mental illness exists in all cultural groups; culture in turn may determine the form in which it appears.

Today, our theories both in psychiatry and anthropology are considerably more sophisticated than those of Daniel Tuke in the last century; our methods include specialized teams of researchers and interview schedules which have been meticulously refined for cross-cultural use. But, despite our progress in theory and methodology, we are left with some of the same concerns voiced in the last century. Mental illness rates are apparently rising in our society, possibly because of changing definitions and methods (13), but rising suicide and crime rates indicate that some of the increase is real. And, to parallel Tuke's concern with the role of deprivation in producing mental illness in the lower classes, twentieth-century studies have shown repeatedly that the highest mental illness rates are in the lowest socioeconomic classes (14).

But, unlike those previously concerned with the interrelations between culture and mental illness, we find ourselves living on a shrinking planet inhabited by more than four billion persons; transcultural psychiatrists find it almost impossible to locate isolated, discrete groups to study. The accelerated rate of change accompanying the technological revolution—fantastic achievements in communications, the emergence of the developing countries, sprawling urbanization, and the centralization of power in the dominant nations—is spreading a veneer of homogeneity over most of our globe. But beneath this thin layer, we find that differing cultural groups may be squeezed into a few blocks of an inner city ghetto. In Miami, for example, Dr. Hazel Weidman (personal communication, 1975) can study a number of subcultural groups living in close proximity in the inner city. Moreover, certain mental illnesses—previously considered exotic—have become visible. These illnesses require description so that they will be recognized by the general physician, most likely a middle-class American without training in the cultural factors underlying the cause and manifestations of various psychiatric and medical illnesses. Sometimes the ill persons require treatments delivered by indigenous or native healers; exorcism and dehexing take place in modern hospitals in the United States. Thus, one critical task for cultural psychiatry is the propagation of the concept that Western society encompasses a collection of subcultures and that it is necessary both to describe culture-specific symptoms and syndromes and to discover effective modes of therapy.

In addition to recognizing the existence of subcultural groups and their variable manifestations of mental disorder, cultural psychiatry is challenged by the problems of acculturation as these groups are subjected to accelerated social-change processes. Alexander Leighton (15) described the problem of acculturation vividly and poignantly in his short essay, "Cosmos in the Gallup City Dump." In his early studies with the Navajo Indians, he found that those who lived on the "septic fringe" and were bombarded by the rapid forces of acculturation demonstrated many symptoms of psychiatric disorder. He states: "... personalities being formed in such culturally confused and depriving circumstances were heavily exposed to noxious influences—according to any psychodynamic theory from Freud to the common sense psychiatry of Adolf Meyer." Subsequent studies of other Indian groups, Eskimos, and the survivors of Hiroshima showed that: "... order in the environment, or at least the resources to create that order, was essential to the human psyche. Without this it seemed that man quickly becomes alien to himself and prone to the conditions he calls psychiatric disorder." Thus, there is an urgent need for cultural psychiatrists, with their awareness of the toll exacted from individuals as America's subcultural groups are thrown deeper into the melting pot.

A culture's "design for living" may be pathogenic. As Wallace (12) points out, "... human instincts are usually gratified, when they are gratified, in a cultural medium; but it is also true that human instincts are frustrated, when they are frustrated, in a cultural medium" (p. 223). Somers (16), in her recent article in *The New England Journal of Medicine*, asserts: "For a considerable proportion of American children and youth, the 'culture of violence' is now both a major health threat and a way of life." She cites evidence that the social causes of death—motor vehicle accidents, suicides, and homicides—are increasing at a rapid rate for the age group 15–24. Mortality from motor vehicle accidents in that age group rose 16 percent between 1963 and 1973. The suicide rate for ages 15–24 more than doubled between 1950 and 1973 to reach a new height of 10.6 per 100,000. And, in 1972, 17 percent of all homicide victims were young people in the age group 20–24. Murder is the fastest growing cause of death in the United States.

Although Somers believes that epidemiologic studies are needed to determine the multiple causes of these alarming facts, she indicts television as a pernicious influence. Television socializes our children and informs, educates, and diverts all of us. It transmits our cultural legacy; the medium is also the message. Strickland (17) states: "Between the ages of 5 and 15, the average American child will view the killing of more than 13,000 persons on television." Furthermore, the massive amount of violence portrayed daily, shows murder, rape, and other crimes occurring in an everyday life setting—probably adding to their impact and contributing to violence as a way of life. Thus, cultural psychiatry's concerns are not limited to exotic syndromes, transcultural comparisons, and acculturation, but also involve the growing number of tragedies of everyday life in modern America.

Another frontier for cultural psychiatry is the increasing number of epidemics of mental illness since World War II. In a definitive article, "Mental Epidemics: A Review of the Old to Prepare for the New," Robert Markush (18) described 33 epidemics of mental disorder that have occurred since 1950.

Modern psychiatry's relative neglect of contagion is surprising in view of the clinical evidence of *folie à deux* or *trois* and the "madness of crowds." A far-reaching type of contagion involves the possibility that the stimulus for rioting and disruption, such as that occurring in America's cities in the late 1960's, was spread through the news media. As Taylor and Hunter (19) explain: "It often requires the adoption of a particular idea by a pluralistically stirred group before the accumulated emotions can be freely expressed. This idea will then appear to have been 'infectious' and to have aroused 'collected emotions'" (p. 837).

In his classic work, *The Epidemics of the Middle Ages*, Hecker (20) described the massive outbreaks of "mental plagues," which were caused in part by cultural factors such as the corruption of morals following the Black Death and the social disorder accompanying the transition to modernity in Europe in the sixteenth and seventeenth centuries. He believed that the strange diseases which became epidemic were spread by morbid sympathy, "on the beams of light—on the wings of thought."

When we consider the problems presented by the commingling of subcultural groups in our urban sprawl, acculturation, our contemporary "culture of violence" and the possible influence of television, Hecker's words from the last century, "on the beams of light—on the wings of thought," heighten our sense of urgency.

We have presented only a few of the serious issues confronting cultural psychiatry—not in the future, but today in our complex, rapidly changing world where man's cultures are being forced together, hastily, without planning, and with an outcome yet to be determined. But, hopefully, the cultures which have now spread to the four, no longer distant, corners of the earth will survive in peaceful commensalism.

REFERENCES

1. Burrows, G.M. *In Inquiry into Certain Errors Relative to Insanity; and Their Consequences; Physical, Moral, and Civil.* London: Thomas and George Underwood, 1820.
2. Halliday, A. *A General View of the Present State of Lunatics and Lunatic Asylums in Great Britain and Ireland, and in Some Other Kingdoms.* London: Thomas and George Underwood, 1828.
3. Esquirol, J.E. A treatise on insanity. In: *Documentary History of Psychiatry*, ed. C.E. Goshen. New York: Philosophical Library, 1967.
4. Kroeber, A.L., and Kluckhohn, C. *Culture: A Critical Review of Concepts and Definitions.* New York: Vintage Books, 1952.
5. Tuke, C.H. *Insanity in Ancient and Modern Life.* London: Macmillan, 1878.
6. Róheim, G. Psycho-analysis and anthropology. In: *Psycho-Analysis Today: Its Scope and Function*, ed. S. Lorand. New York: Covici-Friede, 1933.
7. Malinowski, B. *Magic, Science and Religion and Other Essays.* New York: Doubleday Anchor Books, 1954.
8. Eisenberg, L. The future of psychiatry. *Lancet*, December 15, 1973.
9. Wallace, A.F.C. Science of human behavior: Contribution of the socio-cultural sciences, In: *Comprehensive Textbook of Psychiatry/II*, 2nd ed., Vol. 1, eds. A.M. Freedman, H.I. Kaplan, and B.J. Sadock. Baltimore: Williams & Wilkins, 1975.
10. Eaton, J.W., and Weil, R.J. *Culture and Mental Disorders.* New York: Free Press, 1955.
11. Kluckhohn, C. *Mirror for Man: The Relation of Anthropology to Modern Life.* New York: McGraw-Hill, 1949.
12. Wallace, A.F.C. *Culture and Personality*, 2nd ed. New York: Random House, 1970.

13. Dunham, H.W. Community psychiatry: The newest therapeutic band-wagon. *Arch. Gen. Psychiat.*, 12: 303–313, 1965.
14. Dohrenwend, B.P., and Dohrenwend, B.S. *Social Status and Psychological Disorder: A Casual Inquiry.* New York: Wiley, 1969.
15. Leighton, A. Cosmos in the Gallup City Dump. In: *Psychiatric Disorder and the Urban Environment,* ed. B.H. Kaplan. New York: Behavioral Publications, 1971, pp. 4–12.
16. Somers, A.R. Violence, television and the health of American youth. *New Eng. J. Med.*, 294(15): 811–817.
17. Strickland, S. Who ought to do what about TV violence? Presented at a meeting of the Women's National Democratic Club, Washington, D.C., Februry 18, 1975.
18. Markush, R. *Mental Epidemics: A Review of the Old to Prepare for the New.* Rockville, Md.: Public Health Reviews, 1973.
19. Taylor, F.K., and Hunter, R.C.A. Observations of a hysterical epidemic in a hospital ward: Thoughts on the dynamics of mental epidemics. *Psychiat. Quart.*, 32: 821–839, 1958.
20. Hecker, J.F.C. *The Epidemics of the Middle Ages.* B.G. Babington, Trans., 3rd ed. Completed by the author's treatise on *Child-Pilgrimages*, London: Trübner & Co., 1859.

Index